PERSISTENCE OF VISION

A *portrait of Mother Stanislaus Leary*

by Margaret Brennan SSJ

Persistence of Vision: a portrait of Mother Stanislaus Leary by Margaret Brennan SSJ

© 2005 by the Sisters of St. Joseph of Rochester. All rights reserved.

Quotations
p. 56, Jay P. Dolan, *The American Catholic Experience*, University of Notre Dame Press, ©1992. Used with permission of the publisher.
p. 67 Edward Kantowicz "Schools and Sisters", *Corporation Sole,* University of Notre Dame Press, ©1983 pp 260-263. Used with permission of the publisher.

All quotations originally from the archives of the Diocese of Rochester, Diocese of Buffalo, (including quotation from *The Catholic Union and Times* on p.131), Sisters of St. Joseph Concordia, Sisters of St. Joseph LaGrange, Archives, and Sisters of St. Joseph of Wichita are used with permission.

Photograph credits:
p. 5,16,23,40,51,60,76,78,82,85,88,117,134,148,196,198 Archives, Sisters of St. Joseph of Rochester, New York.
p.35,103,193 Archives, Diocese of Rochester, New York.
p.159 Archives, Sisters of St. Joseph of Concordia, Kansas.
p.187 Sisters of St. Joseph of LaGrange, Illinois. p.6 Ontario County Historical Society.
All photographs used with permission.

ISBN 1-59196-876-3

Printed in the U.S.A. by InstantPublisher.com

Acknowledgements: I wish to acknowledge gratefully the following people for their assistance in the preparation of this book:

First, the archivists and historians who generously shared their time and materials with me: Bonaventure Hill CSJ and Agnes Springer CSJ of LaGrange; Liberata Pellerin CSJ of Concordia; Louise Hune CSJ and Eileen Quinlan CSJ of Wichita; Dorothy Loeb RSM and Jane Hasbrouck RSM of the Rochester Regional Community of the Sisters of Mercy; Rev. William Graf, Barbara Wyand RSM, Rev. Robert McNamara and Robert Vogt of the Diocese of Rochester; Rev. Walter Kern of the Diocese of Buffalo, Mary Ann Butler SSJ and Suzanne Rodriguez SSJ of Buffalo; Patricia Byrne CSJ of Baden, Margaret Quinn CSJ of Brentwood; and our own Jeanne Agnes SSJ and Kathleen Urbanic of Rochester, without whose expertise and research support this story could never have been completed.

Dr. Margaret Susan Thompson of Syracuse University encouraged me to tell the story; Dr. Michael Tomlan of Cornell University helped me try (even if unsucessfully) to puzzle out the mystery of the "mystery house"; Mary John Van Atta SSJ shepherded the project in its beginnings, and Barbara Staropoli SSJ in its completion, giving me the freedom to work and the resources to do the research.

Rev. William H. Shannon, Beatrice Ganley SSJ, Bishop Matthew Clark and Rev. Robert McNamara were gracious in their reading and critiquing the manuscript.

My deepest thanks to Mary Anne Turner SSJ whose skill, patience and expertise created the cover and final formatting design of this book.

Persistence of vision is a visual phenomenon. Because the retina retains a still image for a fraction-of-a-second, consecutive, separate, and rapidly-presented images overlap and meld into one, making them seem to **move** in a fluid, life-like pattern.

Contents

Preface
Pictures: The Portrait

BACKLIGHTING: 1854 - 1867

Chapter 1	Ready for Anything	1
Chapter 2	A Question of Power	10
Chapter 3	No Doubt of the Needs	25

TIME EXPOSURES: 1868 - 1879

Chapter 4	The Best and Ablest of Friends	38
Chapter 5	The Old Balancing Act	55
Chapter 6	Ordinary Time	66
Chapter 7	Days of Miracles	80

THE DARKROOM: 1880 - 1884

Chapter 8	Wholehearted, Unquerying Children	94
Chapter 9	For Reasons Best Known to Himself	110
Chapter 10	If You Will Just Leave Me Alone	126
Chapter 11	They Are Not Here	142

THE DEVELOPING IMAGE: 1884 - 1900

Chapter 12	What the Past Has Made Us	154
Chapter 13	The Dust From My Feet	165
Chapter 14	In a Borrowed Grave	175

A Collage : The Rest of the Picture   183

PREFACE

Histories can be deceiving.

Eyewitness accounts are limiting. Grown siblings often have very different takes on the same childhood incident; investigators know that accident witnesses can contradict each other; perspective is personal.

Autobiography and "as-told-to"s run the risk of being distorted by the subject's lenses; third person narratives are laid open for error by the intrusion of author interpretation.

Even "pure" scholarly history is not all that pure. Layers of research and analysis cannot totally objectify a time, a place, a character, an incident from the prejudices or special interests of the historian.

Histories are deceiving because they are about people, and there is no mystery more compelling and complicated than the mystery of one human life.

When I set out to write this story, my task seemed straightforward and simple: I was to find out what I could about a woman who had been the first superior of our religious order in Rochester from 1868-1882, Mother Stanislaus, née Margaret Leary. She had always been a shadowy figure in our history. We knew that she had been replaced by the bishop under painful circumstances and had left us to found more congregations of Sisters of St. Joseph in the Midwest. My job was to find out what happened, what were the circumstances of her removal. I was to settle the speculation once and for all. That was what I set out to find.

I half-expected to discover a spunky pre-feminist Hollywood-style nun who stood up to a mean bishop in the dear dead days beyond recall, or at least a pious sufferer ennobled by her humiliations, an example to us all. What I found was quite different. Somewhere along the way her story got tangled up with the other stories: of ambitious priests and autocratic bishops; of a system that kept nuns in a paradoxical position of unusual freedom and unconscious servitude; of the power of friendship to build up and tear down; of the uses of convention, power and even religion to hold women to their traditional roles; of the lives of immigrants, pioneers, orphaned children, failed aristocrats, workhouse inmates, convent school girls; of prelates trying, through education and law, to put firm limits on a church growing restive in a hostile Yankee society; of women who, though they seemed worlds apart from us, were the selfsame under the skin.

When I untangled the pieces the woman I found was more a mystery than ever, complex in motive, unpredictable in behavior, with equal parts of fragility and toughness, shrewdness and simplicity. She was circumscribed and defined by her times, as we all are, and can only be discovered before the moving, changing, illusory scrim of nineteenth century America. Though the Catholic Church was a definite subculture of that society, and religious women a sub of that subculture, the lives of these women had an impact that is only now being seriously appreciated and studied.

The irony is not lost on students of American church history that women, by far the larger group of church-goers, the mothers and teachers of the faith for generations of Catholic men, are all but left out of most studies of 19th century Catholicism.

Women religious made the Catholic school system work; they created and operated health care systems; they insisted on accepting people of other religions in their academies and hospitals, predating ecumenism, often the only visible sign of goodwill among the religions in an area; they picked up the pieces of failing social welfare systems by their work with orphans, immigrants, minorities and the urban poor. It is impossible to think of an American Church without them or of the evolution of American women without them.

But somewhere their stories got lost, as did the stories of pioneer women and women who quietly integrated men's professions. Their lives were largely hidden even if their works caused public ripples that reach into our own time.

It is time, now, to tell the stories that will teach us where we came from, our common ground.

This is one of them.

MKB   2005

A PORTRAIT

In 2003 the Rochester Sisters of St. Joseph sold our motherhouse and built a new one on the back half of our property. Lovely as it is, we still mourn the old house, now turned into a college academic center. An imposing English Tudor Gothic brick structure, typical of so many religious houses built in the early decades of this century, it stood on 120 acres of wooded and landscaped land in an affluent suburb of Rochester, New York. Set back, secluded, very private, it provided a beautiful retreat from the outside world, even in modern days when nuns believe that their place is in communion with, not separation from, the world.

When I entered the convent in the mid-1950s, I was sure that it would withstand even a nuclear attack.

By the mid-1980s the inside had become more visitor-friendly than it once was. Quiet carpeting covered the tiles in the corridors, where once clumsy teenage novices were taught the secrets of gliding soundlessly on hard-waxed floors. Talk and laughter filtered through the silences. The *Cloister* signs were long gone--no more mysterious, forbidden places. The dining room, colorful and restful, bore no resemblance to the stern and sterile refectory of earlier days. Original paintings and photographs waited to be admired on every wall.

All of the renovation that had been done had been directed toward gentling, softening, humanizing, home-making the place. But no matter how complete the change, this house could always evoke in me the feeling of a time, a spirituality, an attitude that I usually think of as gone. Being there was revisiting a family homestead and sensing the presence of ancestors. It was in the walls, poured into the concrete, baked into the bricks, carved into the stones. I have no doubt that new generations of college students will sense these presences in the years to come, even if they don't understand quite what they are.

In the front parlor of that place the visitor was surrounded by portraits: nine portraits of our major superiors, hung chronologically, ringing the room. They represented time from 1868 until the end of the twentieth century. One priest I know always called them "The Supremes".

Most of the women in the portraits were familiar to me. I had known them in one way or another. Some I had met. Their faces triggered in me some memory, some incident, some snip of my life. Some, I had only heard about from those who knew them long ago, before I was born. The older Sisters spoke of them with reverence, as they might of saints. Time and distance lend charm.

The first was a mystery to everyone. There is no one now living who remembers her. Her history with us had always been tinted with a sepia cast, never clear black and white. This was Mother Stanislaus. Margaret Leary. Her portrait hung behind the door. One had to search her out.

There was a time when she was not acknowledged at all; there was a time when she was spoken of in whispers, as though there were some vague scandal, some haze about her life with us. In the liberating 1970s and '80s we had started talking about her again. Someone had found her portrait, and she had taken her place on the wall with the other "Supremes."

The portrait is large, slightly fuzzy from the enlarging process, but amazingly clear for the original technology. I think it was taken around 1881, just before "the troubles."

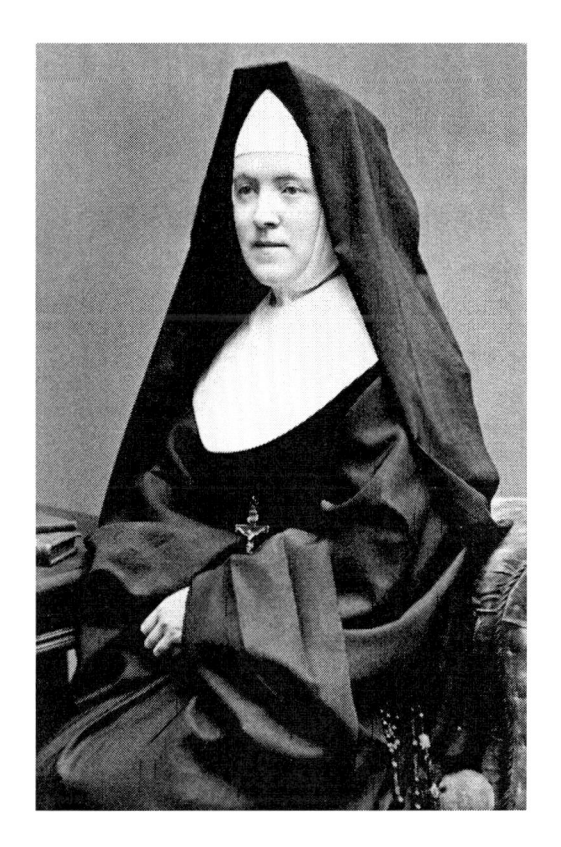

Portrait of Mother Stanislaus Leary

  They say that those with a sensitive eye can read photographs as they might read a diary. Psychologists have used old photos in treating patients, coaxing out long-repressed details, reading old relationships in family pictures: *Why was she looking off while all the rest were attentive to the camera? Why doesn't he touch anyone when all the others are touching? What is the secret of the diffident tilt of the head or the disheveled blouse or the angry stare?*

  Here she looks young, younger than the others on the wall. She is fair-skinned, with light lashes and brows that suggest a redhead or a strawberry blonde. Her hair, of course, is covered by starched white linen and black veiling which she has draped rather dramatically over her right shoulder. *Nice touch, Maggie, I think.*

She does not smile, but one senses the presence of a smile if the photographer would let her, if her dignity would let her, if society would let her. She sits stiffly in the velvet chair, her left hand falling awkwardly from the layers of serge sleeve. Her hand is rough and veined, used to plain work. It is only this hand that gives her forty years away.

My knowing her begins and ends in this picture. In between are theories, diaries, pamphlets and books ; ledgers, annals and stuffy reports; letters, blueprints and property deeds; papers, photos, rumors and facts; librarians, historians, architects and archivists; government documents, memory and tradition; bitterness, brilliance and betrayals

My finger moves from word to blurry word in her diary. Her prose is awkward, words forced from a reluctant pen, brief in pained recalling:

It is a painful experience to recall the particulars of a lifetime marked by sufferings neither few nor small--the loss of one dear relative after another and all my fortune.

Her *fortune*?

and the mental struggles that have filled up each sad interval. It is moreover an undertaking of no small difficulty to one unused to composition to prepare a work for the press

For the *press*?

...nor is it without extreme reluctance that I can bring myself to make reference to those from whom during a long period of years I have been on the most friendly terms and received unvarying kindness.

I hold a brittle letter in my hand. I hold it as I would a holy relic or an antique vase. I know that the faded words are hers, in her own hand, so long ago. I feel that if I look at it harder, if I concentrate I can touch her spirit and learn. I open a ledger page that has not been touched in a hundred years. I rifle through bills and receipts, my fingertips smudged by greasy dust. Goods and services delivered by men long dead.

Will someone, sometime, in a hundred years or so, do the same for any of us? And will they be able to reach beneath the surface of our words, our paper trails, our computer disks, our public images or our myths and find the human part of us that survives?

1 READY FOR ANYTHING

They give themselves to all the works of mercy; they take charge of free schools, hospitals, asylums for foundlings, or for the aged; they may look after prisoners, attend on the poor and the sick in their homes, take care of the infected -- they are ready for anything.

Countess Felicite de Duras, writing to Bishop Rosati of St. Louis, recommending the Sisters of St. Joseph for his diocese.

Even today an overland trip in December from St. Louis to western New York would be risky. The snows of the Great Lakes' southern shores are the stuff of legends. A storm can come up out of nowhere, swirling with "lake effect" white-outs, stranding cars, paralyzing commerce, leaving even snow-ready cities like Buffalo and Rochester at a temporary standstill. Travelers take a chance on such a journey. In 1854 it must have been brutal.

On December 3 of that year four women boarded a boat on the Mississippi that would take them to Alton,

Illinois. Though indistinguishable in their bonnets, flowing skirts and dark capes, they were Catholic Sisters from Carondelet, Missouri, missionaries bound for a small town in what is now known as the Finger Lakes region of New York State. The Sisters of St. Joseph had come to Missouri from Lyons, France only twenty years before, and had already sent out small groups of Sisters like this throughout the Midwest and the East. A bishop would hear of them, request some help, and off they would go, often with total ignorance of the place they might end up.

Religious Sisters did not wear habits when they traveled in the mid nineteenth century. Anti-Catholic, anti-foreign, anti-Irish sentiments of the Know-Nothings were high. Sisters never knew whom they might meet on a long journey, or how insulting and even dangerous such a confrontation might be. Frightening incidents had erupted around the country: riots, street violence, Catholic churches bombed and convents burned. It seemed best to avoid trouble.

They arrived in Alton that evening; by midnight they were perched in a drafty wooden railroad car headed across Illinois to Chicago. The train was cramped and crowded, lit by one or two candles on either end of the car. A wood-burning stove heated the space and there was little ventilation. Bad springs, uneven tracks, bumpy terrain and the not-so-swift speed of twenty-five miles per hour made for a challenging ride in the best of weather. This was an unusually frigid December.

And then there was the snow. The train was forced to stop several times during what should have been a short trip. Squalls, drifts and build-up on the tracks outside; stifling air and freezing feet inside.

It was late the next day when they finally chugged into Chicago, and late into the dark night by the time the tracks were cleared again, so they could head east in the thick snowfall. There was plenty of time to think, if they were wakeful, to talk softly to each other- *Don't attract attention* - to voice their worries - *What if we are stranded? Will there be anyone to meet us when we get there?*- to calm each other's fears. There was plenty of time to let sleep take over, to try to forget their frozen feet, to save their energy for tomorrow. Tomorrow meant another day's journey to Buffalo, trying to endure the boredom in that airless car, too numb to be excited.

By December 7 they were finally and firmly on their last miles. But the weather for which Rochester is world-renowned stopped them one last time. It would be hours, they were told, before they could clear the fast-falling snow from the tracks.

The four, Sisters Francis Joseph Ivory, Agnes Spencer, Theodosia Hageman and novice Petronilla Roscoe, huddled against the wind as they stepped from the train. One of them, Agnes, knew the worst: the money, that they had thought would be more than enough when they left St. Louis, was gone. The others -- exhausted, disoriented, irritable -- only thought of the next step, the next moment, as they looked around the station, down the empty, snowy streets of this unfamiliar city. One of them spotted a cross, the sign of a church, in the distance. Bag and baggage, they started to walk.

The Sisters of Charity had a home for orphans at Rochester's St. Patrick's Church. When the four soggy travelers knocked at their door, the Sisters welcomed them, gave them rest, food and conversation and (when Agnes admitted they had used up all their funds) money for the final hours of the journey. Sr. Francis Joseph was delighted to recognize one of the Charity Sisters, an old school friend from Missouri. They were astounded to meet here, by chance, halfway across the country.

The tracks were clear in a few hours and they

stepped into the stuffy car, ready now for the last lap. The train pulled into the tiny Canandaigua station on the evening of December 7th.

Once again: get up; gather your bundles; make your way out of the stifling car into the flinty snow; accustom your eyes to the darkness and your skin to the breath-stopping cold. It had become a familiar routine in these days, but it would be different this time. They were home.

A dark, bundled figure waved to them. Mr. Cocheran, a railroad official, had come to fetch them. Father O'Connor, he explained, had been summoned on a sick call. They walked the short distance to the priest's house on Pleasant Street, where a welcoming housekeeper sat them down for hot food, and let them politely collapse in a real bed.

The next day they met the pastor, a young man, his head slightly tilted, his longish hair flying, grinning, looking them over with a lazy left eye. Sister Francis Joseph recalled many years later that "he gave a genuine welcome of real old times (and) put us completely at home. From that day his kindness never failed."[1]

County Clare native Edmund O'Connor knew what he wanted. He had been appointed pastor of St. Mary's within a year of his ordination in 1848. Almost at once he had begun a boys' school in the basement of the church, engaging three laymen as teachers. It was not long before he began nudging his bishop to find some Sisters to take it over. Here they were.

He walked them over to Saltonstall Street, to the house that would become the first house of the Sisters of St. Joseph in New York State. Within a short time it would become a, boarding academy, free day school, orphanage, medical dispensary, novitiate, home.

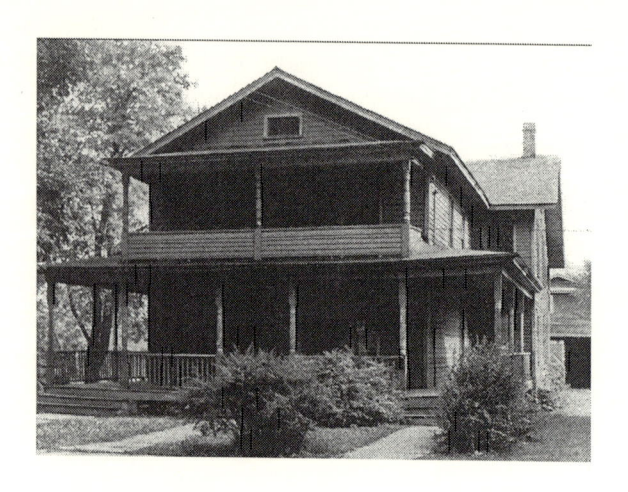

The house on Saltonstall Street

In 1854 all of Western New York was one diocese, with Buffalo its See City. Bishop John Timon had known the Sisters of St. Joseph when he was a Lazarist missionary in the Mississippi Valley and the Southwest frontier. When Edmund O'Connor requested some religious to help his growing parish, Timon wrote to the community in Carondelet, asking them to make a foundation in his diocese.

Sister Agnes Spencer was a sensible choice to lead such a group. She had worked in two new foundations in the eight years she had been in the community. Agnes had a real missionary temperament. She seemed fearless, creative and hard-working. She would be needing these qualities.

The Saltonstall Street house was roomy enough for four Sisters. The spacious yard gave breathing room and thick shrubs offered privacy from curious eyes. But the house soon became the center of their ministry and the walls closed in.

They took over the boys' school in the church basement. Within a month they had set up their own home as a boarding school for "poor girls of good character," a select academy that would help to pay for the free school, and an orphanage. Agnes, who had skills as an herbalist, set up a small dispensary in the house as well, and the poor of the town came to her for basic medical treatment. How these rather disparate works went on in the same household, along with their own religious community life, is a mystery. Active religious in America learned early on the tension between the demands of their ministry and their religious rule.

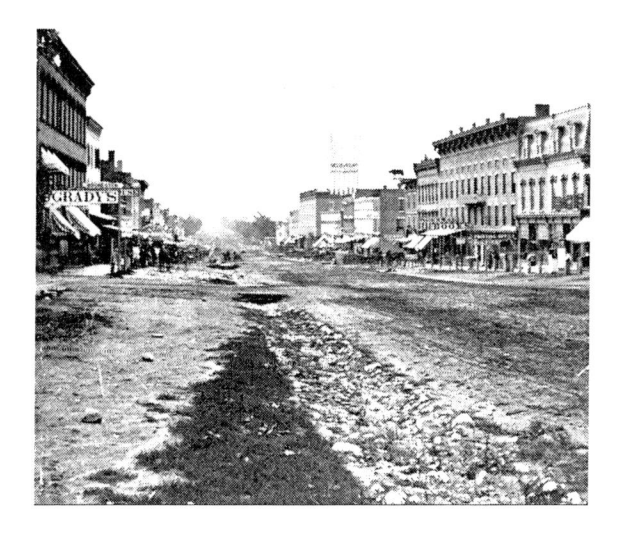

Main Street, Canandaigua in the 1860s

    Evidently they tried to do too much too soon. The academy tuition was not the strong source of income they had expected, and the Sisters literally went begging in town for money to keep things going. Some of the parishioners at St. Mary's were appalled; they suggested that the Sisters close up and withdraw, since they could not seem to support themselves and the parish was struggling financially. The Sisters' poverty in their midst was an embarrassment.

Edmund O'Connor had waited too long for these women to let them go, so with Irish passion and persuasion he appealed for assistance from some wealthy Catholic Canandaiguans, at the same time mollifying his worried and doubtful parishioners. A core group of men-of-means agreed to provide financial support where it was needed. The Sisters, their fate decided by powerful men, remained.

Now that the original four had established themselves, and it seemed clear that they would stay, Agnes asked for help. Sisters were sent from St. Louis and Philadelphia to join them. Among the new arrivals was a young Sister from Philadelphia, Sister Baptista Hanson.

Bishop Timon liked what he saw in the Canandaigua group and wanted to increase their visibility in the diocese. He had an agenda of his own for them- a school for the deaf in Buffalo. The Sisters of St. Joseph were known for their work with the deaf, both in France and in the Missouri missions. The superior of the Philadelphia Sisters, Mother St. John Fornier, happened to be an old friend of Timon's. He wrote to her, begging for Sisters to do this work in his diocese:

Already I thank God we have your good Sisters in my diocese, but I wish to see them in the Episcopal City...I have a large lot in a beautiful situation which was given to me to found a Deaf and Dumb Asylum...My thoughts have long been turned to your Society for this, and I wished to see what help I could expect and whether you have any Sisters who are able to teach the deaf and dumb. If your community would not undertake the deaf and dumb asylum, I would still wish them to teach and fill other offices of charity in Buffalo.[2]

While he was at it, Timon also put in a word for his friend, Bishop John Loughlin of Brooklyn, who was looking for a community of Sisters for his diocese. The trading of nuns was the order of the day.

Mysterious conflict and a "trade"

Something was going on in Canandaigua. Only shadows and traces of the problem survive, but whatever troubles the Sisters were having, Sister Baptista Hanson seemed to be in the midst of them. In June of 1856 Timon wrote again to Mother St. John, thanking her for her interest in the Buffalo community, agreeing to some sort of exchange of Sisters, and noting, cryptically, that "Now all is quiet; all seem to be doing their best; it is better to make no change until after the end of Studies."[3]

Father O'Connor, typically, was more blunt. In August he pleaded with Mother St. John to send a Sister deSales in exchange for Baptista:

When a man is in want, you will admit that he must ask, and that from those who can give. Some time ago I requested of you to give me a Sister in exchange for Sister Baptista, This you refused and assigned your reasons which were sufficiently strong...Now it is the wish of Sr. Baptista to return to Philadelphia. It is M[other] A[gnes].'s wish and also mine and that from conscientious motives. You see, you have no excuse now, no blame can be attached to you...I will go south here to Phil. I wish to get in exchange Sr. deSales who fought so hard to come with me. Baptista I like much, I would not part with her if I could, but I tell you as a secret that her salvation is in danger by staying here.[4]

Baptista's soul was spared whatever dire consequences O'Connor hinted at. By August 12, 1856, Sisters Baptista and Theodosia had their official obedience (walking papers!) from Bishop Timon, appointing them "to begin...a house of your order in the diocese of Brooklyn."[5] Baptista had been traded.

Two months later the community in Canandaigua turned a corner. Whatever internal problems they had been experiencing, they had a fresh start. Two young women from Corning were received as postulants on October 15, 1856.

Bishop Timon had personally steered Margaret Leary and Margaret Donovan to this new religious community. Their entrance meant the opening of a novitiate, with the assurance that this was now a genuine foundation of the Sisters of St. Joseph in his diocese. There had been many comings and goings, transfers and exchanges in the two year since they had arrived from St. Louis. The establishment of a novitiate gave stability and a sure future. It would be better all around. The exchanges of Sisters with Philadelphia and other foundations would continue until Timon's death in 1867, but Buffalo now had its own training ground and independence.

For Western New York it meant the start of a group of women whose work would weave itself into the fabric of that society.

For the Sisters of St. Joseph, it meant an expansion into one of the fastest growing urban areas in the country - a chance to grow, to extend their ministry, to make a difference.

For fifteen year old Margaret Leary it marked a journey that would span half the continent and take her from the Civil War to the Gilded Age.

2   A QUESTION OF POWER

Behold, you are dead to the world. Are you satisfied?

Reception Ceremony, Sisters of St. Joseph

It would be a great charity if we could have at least one trusty Sister to be Superior.

Bishop John Timon to Mother St. John Fornier

Born in New York City on August 15, 1841, Margaret Leary was the daughter of Irish immigrant Michael Leary and New Yorker Ann O'Connor.[1] Only fragments of her early life survive. In her diary, written toward the end of her life, she writes very briefly that they moved to Corning, New York when she was about seven and that her father, a merchant, died shortly after that move. Corning's first village census, taken in 1849, lists an Ann Leary as head of a family of seven. Michael had died, leaving Ann to care for their son and five daughters. Nellie, the youngest, was only weeks old.[2]

Corning, New York was still a small farming community in the late 1840's. With the immigrant explosion, it was growing fast; the largest immigrant population by far was Irish. If the shock of coming from New York City to this place was great, at least the Learys would have felt at home among "their own." They would have felt the same wave of intolerance as the other Irish Catholics in New York State at that time. And they would have suffered from the devastation of fire and flood that hit Corning in 1856 and 1857.

A few months before Margaret entered the convent in 1856, two fires swept through the town, burning barns, liveries and businesses, killing livestock, turning stored crops to ashes. The next summer the town was submerged in floods from heavy rains and the overflowing Chemung River, floods that would wash away field crops and family gardens, animals and even small buildings.[3]

And they would have been subject to the same primitive medical care as others in the area. Children were the primary victims of this system, many dying from or permanently weakened by untreated whooping cough, scarlet fever, diarrhea and croup. Margaret Leary's health was always delicate, marked by frequent bouts of unspecified illness that would underpin events in her life and sometimes even determine the course of action she chose to take. It was this vague "delicateness" that prompted her superiors to send her away almost as soon as she entered!

The new "Brides of Christ"

After only four months as postulants, the two Margarets from Corning received the habit on February 14, 1857 in St. Mary's Church in Canandaigua. The event was a novelty for the parishioners, who had never seen a religious reception and were moved by the sight of these two teenagers in bridal gowns and veils, symbols of their new life as "Brides of Christ," being questioned by Bishop Timon about their intentions.

This ceremony remained the reception rite for Sisters of St. Joseph in Rochester (with minor modifications) until well into the 1960's. It exemplifies a spirituality familiar to Catholics raised before Vatican II. Religious life required death to the world, childlike obedience, and the necessity of literally giving up everything to follow Christ. Heavy decisions for sixteen-year-olds! In the ceremony the Bishop tells the postulant:

In order to become a true Sister of St. Joseph, you should, my child, die to the world, to your parents, to your friends, and to yourself and live alone for Jesus Christ.

And she replies:
That is what I desire with all my heart; that the world be nothing more to me and Jesus be my only possession.

He: *Do you desire at once to renounce the world, its vanities and its pomps and to take the poor habit of the Sisters of St. Joseph?*

She: *It is a long time that I have ardently desired it and I beg of you not to defer it any longer.*

He: *I am satisfied to do so, my child, and I desire Mother Superior to receive you into the Congregation, to retrench this superfluity of*

> *hair and divest you of your worldly dress, in order to put on the poor habit you long for with so much ardor.*

He sends her off. She returns in a black habit and veil, now virtually indistinguishable from the other Sisters, anonymous. She will be given a new name and be, from that moment on, a new person. He asks her: *Behold, you are dead to the world. Are you satisfied?*

> She: *Yes...I am quite satisfied. I experience the most perfect joy of heart...I value this above all the goods of the world. These glorious advantages enable me to leave with joy my parents, my friends and all the vanities of the world.*[4]

Margaret Leary had chosen to enter religious life at a time when it would seem that her mother needed her at home. Ann Leary was a young widow with five other children to care for; letting Margaret go must have been a heavy burden for her. However, there was a certain status in a Catholic (especially an Irish Catholic) household in having a priest or nun in the family, so perhaps Ann thought it would bring a blessing to her family. And, after the modest dowry was paid, it also meant one fewer mouth to feed. Whatever the situation, it could not have been easy for her, and must have been a blow when she heard her Margaret answer Bishop Timon that she left her family "with joy"!

Margaret Leary became Sister Stanislaus and Margaret Donovan Sister Anastasia. By the time they were twenty-seven, each would be the major superior of a religious congregation.

Sister Baptista and the new novice

The next two years pose a problem, since there are two believable accounts of Novice Stanislaus' whereabouts. Her act of profession states: "I received the habit in our house of Canandaigua...and afterwards I made my novitiate in the same house...during the space of twelve months, the rest of the time in our house in Buffalo."[5] However, the annals of the Rochester congregation contradict this formal statement:

A change of air was judged necessary for Sr. Stanislaus and following Bishop Timon's advice, Mother Agnes Spencer sent her to Brooklyn where under the loving care of Sr. Baptista Hanson, the young Sister passed the two years of her novitiate."[6]

Sister Baptista Hanson? Brooklyn? A growing city like Brooklyn may not seem the place for a "change of air," but it is not surprising that Sister Stanislaus might have been sent there. Whatever problems the Canandaigua house had worried through in the year before, and whatever Baptista's part in them might have been, Agnes obviously trusted her, confirming her assignment to go with Theodosia to start a new foundation in Brooklyn. The Brooklyn mission was struggling: there were the demands of a new school, the expectations of their Bishop, the adjustments and anxieties of being on their own, of starting something new.

It had been only three years since they had stepped off that snowy train from St. Louis, and Agnes was just beginning to see some stability and future in this new community. It had begun to feel less like a mission outpost and more like a real foundation. Why not help the new group as they had been helped by "loans" from St. Louis and Philadelphia? And why not send Bishop Timon's own protegeé, Margaret Leary, to help out his old friend John Loughlin?

About one thing there is no doubt: Sister Stanislaus and Sister Baptista became close friends. Their friendship would be a source of strength and trouble as the years went on. Young Stanislaus was an eager, empty page to be written on; Baptista was strong and controversial.

More trouble in Canandaigua: the locus of power

In Canandaigua the work flourished, especially at St. Mary's Academy, which attracted a good number of young women whose families wanted them to have the advantage of a European-style education.[7] Because of this, the financial situation had stabilized to the point that Mother Agnes was able to pay on a mortgage for some property.

It is not clear whether this was the Saltonstall Street house or some other property that she wanted for the community's work; in any case, it became the focus of a serious dispute between Agnes and the bishop of Buffalo and the first test of his authority as superior of the Superior!

Power. It always was and always will be a question of the locus of power. John Timon wanted the Sisters of St. Joseph to prosper in his diocese. This community was in demand among American bishops because of the freedom which their rule afforded them to do any work requested by a bishop. There was a specific directive in their rule, naming the local bishop in whatever diocese they found themselves as their highest superior. This was a dream situation for any bishop: free, or at least very cheap, labor by women who were under vow to obey him.

Timon was anxious to have a Mother Superior appointed or elected for the entire district encompassed by his diocese. Mother Agnes had led the group since their arrival. The Sisters seemed satisfied with her, even devoted to her, but the bishop was uneasy. Several young women had joined the community and he had his own ideas about how and where they would serve his diocese. He needed a superior who would cooperate, who would put her Sisters completely at his service.

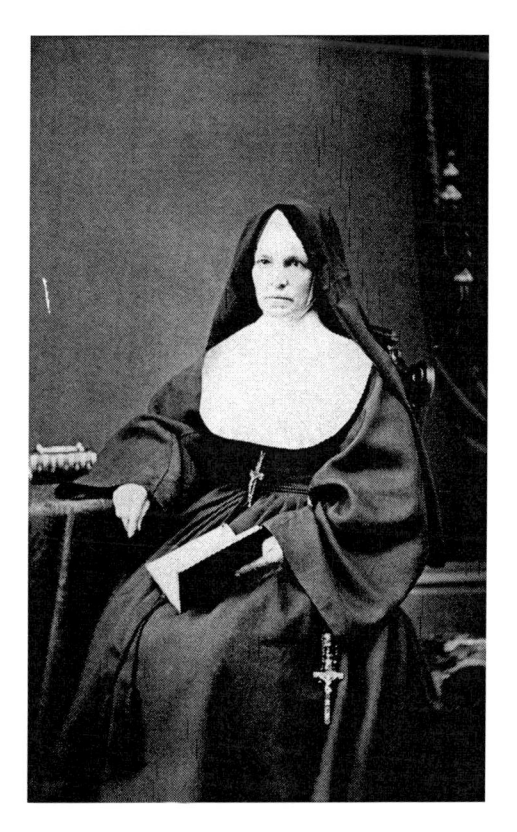

Sister Agnes Spencer

Sister Agnes Spencer's independence was a stumbling block for him. Her self-reliance had made her a good missionary. She knew how to search out needs and respond to them: her little dispensary in Canandaigua; her visiting the sick in their homes; her work with families and the poor in Dunkirk, a little town near Buffalo. She was a visible presence; people knew her and would remember her for years after she left.

But she was not the sort of administrator that Timon wanted for this new community. He decided to let the Sisters decide about their leadership. In 1858 he wrote to Mother St. John in Philadelphia:

> I have seen that much of the suffering comes from doubts about who might be the Mother for this district. Here I have required that all the professed Sisters meet in Buffalo to make three days retreat which I will conduct myself; and then give their votes for Superior of the central house...[8]

To his credit, he did ask for her advice "so that I may know better and better what may be for the good of a Society so dear to me." And so valuable, too, to carry out his plans.

The Sisters evidently voted for Agnes Spencer. Timon seemed to be doubtful about her ability to lead the community and ordered her, three months later, to bring the novitiate from Canandaigua to Buffalo. He himself would give the novices instruction and monitor Agnes' leadership. "Everything depends on Sister Agnes," he wrote Mother St. John, "May God give her the right spirit."[9]

Sister Stanislaus was gathered home from Brooklyn to finish her training with the four or five others who had entered after her. Though novices were rarely privy to the worries and decisions of their superiors, it would have been hard to miss the tension between John Timon and their Reverend Mother. She would learn young about the consequences of crossing a bishop.

It seemed imperative that the main house and novitiate be moved from Canandaigua, where trouble hadn't ceased. Father O'Connor had been stripped of his pastorate at St. Mary's. It could not have been a pleasant affair. Though the reason for his replacement of Edmund O'Connor doesn't survive, Bishop Timon's attitude comes through loud and clear in correspondence with Mother St. John.

It seems that Sister Agnes had taken O'Connor's side against the bishop. She did not have "the right spirit" that John Timon was looking for. Not only was he angered by her friendship with O'Connor, there was also this Canandaigua property to be dealt with. Whatever this property was, he wanted it. It was simple.

Timon's diary from 1859 reveals how quickly things happened:

June 11	*See Sisters of St. Joseph; instruct. Call on Sr. Agnes Spencer to make deed for land at Canandaigua, refuses. Call her again at 2 P.M., refuses. I insist, offer her a mortgage for what she says she has paid. She asks for time, give her till 11 on Monday.*
June 13	*Sr. Agnes refuses, give her till evening, go consult Sr. Julia, ask Agnes her determination, she says she will not submit, but will go. [I] depose her but tell her in the presence of Srs. Anselm and Julia that if she comes before 9 tomorrow and promises to observe the rules, and have them observed I will reverse what I have done, name Sr. Julia in her place.*
June 14	*Sr. Agnes does not come at 4 P.M., go up, find Sisters from Dunkirk, Canandaigua, announce the depositions, name Sr. Julia General Superior...Sr. Agnes retracts.*
June 15	*...Sr. Agnes engages to return and take any position I may give her, tell her that I cannot restore her, but that I will do what I can for her, give her $25.*[10]

The next day he wrote to Mother St. John, telling her that Edmund O'Connor's influence was still felt there, that Sister Agnes had refused to cooperate and that he had "deposed" her.

While he was in Canandaigua he also ordered "one of the Miss Traceys" out of the Canandaigua house.[11] Father O'Connor's nieces, Margaret and Anna Tracey, had been friends of the Sisters since their arrival and there was evidently a lingering bad feeling between Timon and any O'Connor connection. It seems clear that Agnes Spencer paid a price for her loyalty to Edmund O'Connor.

None of this could have been lost on Sister Stanislaus. The scenario would be repeated in her life. She had made her profession of vows in April 1859, in the midst of all the trouble. It was time for her first assignment.

St. Mary of the Lake, Buffalo

Father James Early had asked for Sisters to staff a free school for poor children in his parish, St. Mary's of the Lake in Buffalo. Early was known as an advocate for the poor, especially children. Short, energetic, gifted with a wry sense of humor and an ability to involve others in his projects, he made devoted friends and admirers easily. There was a passion about him that attracted people.

Sister Stanislaus was assigned to St. Mary's. She was only nineteen, but had already had some teaching experience in Brooklyn. At St. Mary's the Sisters lived in three little cottages that had been built on the property of the Deaf-Mute Institute. They taught the children in an old wooden church.

The concept of the free school was dear to John Timon's heart. It was customary for religious communities to run a "select" school or academy along with their schools for the poor. The income from the tuition school supported the free school. Timon resisted this system. There was no select school at St. Mary of the Lake, and the conditions were poor, almost primitive. Food was scarce, Buffalo winters frigid; often there was not enough firewood for both convent and school, so school got the heat. Most of the Sisters were young and resilient. Accounts of those days of deprivation stress the happiness rather than the sacrifice.

It was here that Sister Stanislaus first worked with James Early. Though their friendship would not be cemented until a few years had passed, it would change both their lives.

Sister Julia Littlenecker took over as superior, without benefit of election, and Sister Agnes stayed on for a while. Her presence troubled the bishop, who complained to Mother St. John that Agnes and another Sister were "intriguing" against him:

> They have written to various bishops, without knowledge of S. Julia or of me, to obtain a place. Of course I know not what day they may silently depart. The priest gave Sister Agnes about $500 some time ago. She keeps part in the house and has $300 deposited in Bank in the name of Agnes Spencer. Her sister, S. Augustine, was made superior in Canandaigua. She there keeps up the old spirit. In both places they hold communication with Rev. E. O'Connor. It would be a great charity if we could have at least one trusty Sister to be Superior.[12]

John Timon was not above a bit of sarcasm.

Not long after this, Sister Agnes Spencer went south to Pennsylvania, out of Buffalo's jurisdiction, and started another eastern foundation that would eventually be centered in Erie. This time she had some money.

Mother Agnes Spencer's story is hardly unique in the 19th century American Church. In fact, it was just such disagreements with bishops (often about property; always about power) that caused new foundations to spring up all over the country.

Bishops vie for power over "their" Sisters

Now that Bishop Timon was rid of Agnes Spencer, he turned his attention to another problem with the Sisters of St. Joseph. A movement was underway to reorganize the Sisters of St. Joseph in the United States. According to the plan, the central motherhouse would be at Carondelet, Missouri and the other houses throughout the country would belong to regional provinces, all ultimately governed by Carondelet. That meant, of course, that they would also ultimately be governed by the archbishop of St. Louis rather than by local bishops.

Thus began a power struggle, not among the Sisters, but among the bishops, who did not want "their" Sisters subject to St. Louis. A bishop would not be governed by his peers, nor have his subjects governed by them.

Timon, himself a member of a religious order, had inserted himself into the lives of the religious communities of his diocese. He knew their worth, their potential, their value, if the works he envisioned for the diocese were to be realized. He could not afford to lose this growing congregation to another jurisdiction. He needed absolute authority.

Timon encouraged Mother St. John to remain firm against the movement as well. "God will protect his work," he wrote to her. "Time, too will enable those who press upon you to see that the movement is wrong and will scarcely be encouraged anywhere."[13]

During a retreat he gave to her Sisters in Philadelphia, Timon publicly denounced the plan and urged the community to resist. He had allies in the fight. The bishops of Philadelphia, Wheeling, Toronto, Brooklyn and Hamilton all knew the advantage in having independent groups of women religious in their diocese and joined Timon in his crusade to keep things as they were.

The community in Carondelet drafted a temporary Constitution outlining the provincial plan and the Sisters in Philadelphia wrote another as an independent diocesan congregation. The race was on.

In June of 1862 five North American bishops, in Rome for their regular *ad-limina* visit to the Pope, caucused about getting the Philadelphia rule approved, while the Bishop of Albany lobbied for Carondelet's. Timon wrote to the Philadelphia community:

> As soon as I came to Rome I called upon the Cardinal to obtain the approbation of your rules. It gave me great hope and I gathered the bishops of Philadelphia, of Toronto, Brooklyn and Hamilton and we five have been for some time preparing for the work. I must tell you that the Bishop of Albany says that he is commissioned by St. Louis to get their new rule approved. You must pray and get others to pray. I had my petition for your approbation at least two weeks before Bishop. McClosky could have made his.[14]

Eventually both rules were approved: Albany, New York and St. Paul, Minnesota became provinces of the Carondelet community; the Buffalo community adopted the Philadelphia rule and became an independent diocesan order. Several of the Buffalo Sisters returned to Carondelet, including the superior, Sister Julia.

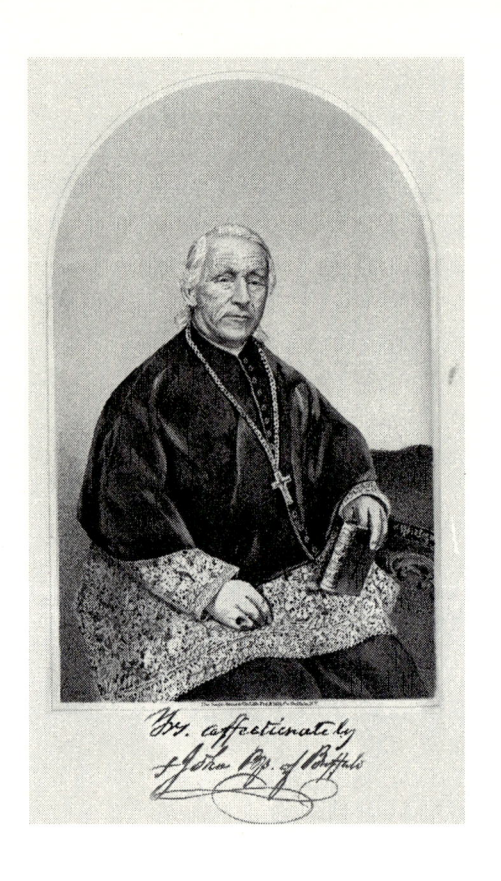

Bishop John Timon

    Timon began once again to negotiate for someone he could count on to lead the shaky group, to help them recover from their losses, and get on with their lives and the work of his diocese. Once again he called on Philadelphia, who sent Sister Magdalen Weber "on loan" to become the new superior of the Buffalo Sisters. There is no record of an election, even though the new rule called for one. Like Sister Julia, Magdalen was a Timon appointee. His control over the young community was secure.
    In 1861 Sister Stanislaus went to Dunkirk to take

the place of Agnes Spencer, who had started the mission three years before. The tension of those days, Agnes' disagreements with the bishop and her eventual replacement are nowhere to be found in the official accounts. We read only that she left and Sister Stanislaus and others continued the work.

At the same time James Early left St. Mary's of the Lake as well, taking the pastorate in another St. Mary's, Canandaigua. His life was becoming more and more woven with the Sisters of St. Joseph.

3 NO DOUBT OF THE NEEDS

> *Among the disastrous consequences of the Civil War was the vast number of children all over the land whom it rendered fatherless and oft-times homeless...(this) was deeply felt in Rochester, N.Y., a city located in the western part of the state on the Genesee River...In the autumn of 1864, the venerable John Timon sent a colony of the Sisters of St. Joseph to open an Asylum for the soldiers' orphans at Rochester.*

Annals, Sisters of St. Joseph of Rochester

The Buffalo diocese embraced the twenty counties of Western New York, from Syracuse to Buffalo, from Canada to the Pennsylvania border. Bishop Timon, once a missionary in the Southwest, traveled hundreds of miles by carriage, by train, by horseback, by boat, even by sleigh to visit parishes, administer sacraments, admonish, and encourage. He seemed to be everywhere.

A former superior in his own religious community, Timon was used to unquestioning obedience. He well knew the inadequacy of much of the priestly training in the United States, and the needs of his largely immigrant flock. He kept a strict eye on priests and people, the virtual pastor in every parish. In spite of his energetic efforts, it became increasingly impossible to keep up the personal contact as the villages grew into towns, the towns into cities.

Early settlers had expected that the village of Canandaigua would grow quickly into a center of trade and industry. Instead it was its neighbor, Rochester, which mushroomed. A port of Lake Ontario, the Genesee River and the Erie Canal, Rochester soon surpassed little Canandaigua.

Rochester Catholics wanted their own diocese. This feeling intensified as the population grew, churches opened and religious communities arrived to help. The Sisters of Mercy, the Christian Brothers, the Religious of the Sacred Heart, the Sisters of Charity, the School Sisters of Notre Dame made their presence and the presence of the Church felt in a decidedly WASP society. Though that society didn't know it, Rochester needed their help. Most of the immigrant population was Catholic; social services were in a sorry state; and the Civil War had come home.

Rochester was not exempt from the xenophobia of the rest of the eastern states. Immigrants, far from being unconditionally welcomed, were often greeted with scorn and even brutality by "native" Rochesterians (who seemed not at all aware that it was the Senecas, not they, who were the natives). Menial, low-paying jobs, poor education, squalid housing and prejudice kept immigrants in their place. They were blamed for crime, denied access to employment, punished for being poor. In other words, it was a time much like our own.

Many, if not most, immigrants were Catholics --

Irish and German, mainly. The Catholic community closed ranks to help them.

Social problems in Rochester: almshouses and orphans

However progressive, sophisticated and humane Rochester may have considered itself, it suffered the same social problems as other growing urban areas of the mid-nineteenth century: epidemic disease, high infant mortality, unemployment, poor medical treatment, contaminated food and water supplies, the realities of families broken or separated by the war. By 1860, one-half of recorded deaths in the city were young children, most of them from the tenements of the immigrant families or from the Almshouse.[1]

Early attempts to address social problems had been too little, too cold. The unemployed begged pennies for food; their wives died in "childbed fever" caused by dirty hands and instruments; their children died of unchecked diseases or survived to run wild and get into trouble.

The county built an almshouse in 1826; before long it was overcrowded. Some vocal citizens quickly grew tired of supporting the (mostly immigrant) poor, insisting that the Almshouse inmates work harder, to save county money. An editorial in the Rochester *Daily Advertiser* declared that "a house of public charity should not become a house of luxury, thus offering to the vicious and idle a reward and a comfortable home."[2]

The truth was that no one was idle. Many of the men were skilled craftsmen who used their skills as carpenters, blacksmiths and masons; some worked the farm. There is even a physician listed in the Almshouse residents' records of the time. Women cleaned houses or worked as seamstresses or servants. The younger children went to school, while the older ones helped their parents.[3]

But the conditions in this place of "charity" were positively Dickensian: disease took whole families at a time; alcoholism and alcohol-related deaths were common, fueling the anti-poor, anti-Irish bias even more, and Almshouse residents were blamed for crime and moral degradation in that most virtuous Yankee city.

Some forward-looking citizens thought that the only hope was in the children. In 1837 a group of women of some means had the idea for a Rochester orphan asylum to rescue the children from the Almshouse. In three years it officially opened.

Around the same time Rochester Catholics were concerned about the fate of Catholic children in the public institutions, where Catholics were denied access to religious services, instruction and sacraments. A movement was begun to raise money for a girls' Catholic orphan asylum. They would start with the little girls. The project began modestly in the back of St. Patrick's Church in 1842.

The Sisters of Charity arrived three years later to take charge. These were the same Sisters, and this the same place that rescued the four snowbound Sisters of St. Joseph on their way to Canandaigua on December 7, 1854. Their lives would cross again.

The war comes home

Western New York was not a battleground of the Civil War but suffered visibly from it. At the war's start, "war fever" took over in Rochester, with displays of patriotism, downtown parades of army recruits, public pleas to preserve the Union. The enthusiasm seemed to cross ethnic lines in a city where those lines had been firmly and sometimes bitterly drawn. On May 3, 1861,

State and Exchange Streets were alive with 20,000 Rochesterians, loud and proud, gathered to send the first wave of local boys off to Elmira. From there they would go to Washington, to protect the capital from attack.

Rochester had been fertile ground for the Union cause. In 1858 William Seward gave his "Irrepressible Conflict" speech in the city's Corinthian Hall. When South Carolina seceded two years later, Rochester residents Susan B. Anthony and Frederick Douglass held a convention in the same place, urging Lincoln to stand firm on the slavery issue. Both had been keeping the abolitionist position before the public for some time, so Rochesterians were well aware of the issues and ready to do what had to be done.

Their enthusiasm was brief. It lasted only until the first casualties began arriving home on the same trains that had taken them south. Lists of the dead grew and many wounded were taken to St. Mary's Hospital, opened in 1867 by Sister of Charity Hieronymo O'Brien.

St. Mary's Hospital was Bishop Timon's pride and joy, and rightly so. The only hospital in Western New York outside of Buffalo, St. Mary's became one of the few examples of religious tolerance in an area where Catholics were so often mistrusted and mistreated. When it opened, a public advertisement assured the people of Rochester that everyone would be admitted, without prejudice or distinction, whatever their belief or unbelief, that patients would have full access to their pastors or ministers, that the poor would be treated gratis.

Public support for the hospital grew as the war wounded were carried home and the Sisters kept their promises. St. Mary's and its hearty foundress, Mother Hieronymo, enjoyed a respect and acceptance in the Rochester community that no cleric had been able to attain.

It soon became apparent that there were other war casualties: young widows and homeless children.

St. Mary's Boys' Home: a haven in the center of the city

Father James Early had been in Canandaigua for only one year. While he was pastor he had remodeled the sanctuary of the church, had become involved with the orphan children, and had become friendly with the Sisters on Saltonstall Street. His pastorate at St. Mary's was mysteriously brief. In 1862 he was reassigned to another St. Mary's - in Rochester. The church was in the very center of the growing city. It was not long before he knew he had to address a clear and present need: a home for boys.

Street boys had become a genuine problem that had increased as the war dragged on. Some were abandoned, some orphaned, some neglected, some escaped to the streets from the hard life in the county Almshouse, some unable to be controlled by widowed mothers. Dependent Catholic boys were sent to St. Joseph's Home in Buffalo, further separating them from families.

The Sisters of Mercy worked with Early at St. Mary's where they conducted a select school for girls, a free school, soup kitchen and a House of Mercy for homeless women. When Early appealed to Bishop Timon for some Sisters to begin a home for boys, Timon approached the Sisters of Mercy. Mother Camillus, the superior, was reluctant to accept an undertaking like this one. Her Sisters were overworked as it was, and their community had been founded to care for women and girls. She felt it would be against their tradition to take on a new work with boys.[4]

Early bought Park House, a two-story brick building on South Street, next to the church. He had worked with the Sisters of St. Joseph in Buffalo and Canandaigua. He asked Bishop Timon for some Sisters from this community, had asked, in fact, for a specific Sister who had been a friend of his in Canandaigua.[5] The community sent, instead, four young Sisters (they were all young in those days!), appointing twenty-four year old Sister Stanislaus Leary as superior of the group. He knew her, of course, from St. Mary's of the Lake, though there is no evidence that they were friends. If Early was disappointed at first, he would soon change his mind.

    Sisters Stanislaus and Xavier Delahunty had been enjoying their work in Dunkirk. Things had begun to ease; they loved the children and the work; they had just moved into a new home. They had no experience in starting a mission from scratch.[6] Along with lay Sisters Clare O'Shea and Martina Hogan they moved into Park House on November 1, 1864. News of their arrival must have been on the street. The first evening there was a knock at their door. On the stoop stood two small boys, asking for shelter.

    There was no doubt of the need. Only months later St. Mary's was home to about thirty five-to-ten-year old boys. A board of trustees, with Father Early and Sister Stanislaus as president and secretary-treasurer, took over the financial responsibility and St. Mary's Boys' Asylum was a going concern.

    There was much to be done to provide home, education, and emotional support for these boys. The Early-Leary team worked well together. He searched out the funds and gave good-natured moral support; she organized their small community to be teachers, advocates, and substitute mothers.

    An editorial in the Rochester *Union and Advertiser* gave the work a public boost three months later:

Among the charities of this city entitled to especial favor and which had received as yet but little attention is the institution on South

Street...St. Mary's Asylum for Orphan Boys. The purpose of the institution is to gather in those boys who, left without parents or guardians, and in indigent circumstances, are left to wander in the world to become in most cases vicious men. Now more than ever should such institutions be fostered when this terrible war is so rapidly multiplying the list of orphans...A visit to the institution on Saturday was gratifying to us. The house, though not yet fully supplied with the furniture required, is provided with nice beds for the boys, with the fuel and food for the time being, and the little fellows seem to be very happy and comfortable. In the school room they are taught all the English studies adapted to children of their age...This orphan asylum will continue to receive boys as they are found neglected, and they will remain there to be instructed and when of suitable age, they will be provided with homes where they can engage in respectable vocations to earn their livelihood. Such an institution commends itself to the public and bespeak for it the attention of the benevolent and the assistance of the public authorities.[7]

Money was always tight, provisions scarce. Rochester lived in a wartime economy, with all of the deprivations that that implies.

Such free advertising from the press could only help. The Genesee River overflowed its banks in March of 1865, flooding the city center. Damaged gas mains left the city dark for days; the New York Central railroad bridge and some of the Erie tracks floated away, stopping rail transportation, and paralyzing a good portion of trade in the city.

The Sisters at St. Mary's Asylum needed help. They were used to simple living, tight belts (or, in their case, cinctures), plain and often small amounts of food, scraping around for money to pay the bills. The boys needed more than St. Mary's could easily provide. The Sisters could not sacrifice good food and hygienic surroundings. They knew stories of the Almshouse, of the spread of disease, the dangers of fire. If they were to continue to take children in, they knew there had to be a firm financial base. Their own resources were few, so they turned to civic authorities.

St. Francis deSales is credited as the author of an old technique for winning people over: "You can catch more flies with a teaspoon of honey than with a barrel of vinegar." Sister Stanislaus (young, pretty, smiling) invited the Board of Education to visit their little school; she welcomed reporters and gave tours; she arranged for a fair to be held downtown, assuring widest visibility, well aware of the emotional impact on potential benefactors of watching little orphan boys sing on the stage of Washington Hall. The teaspoon of honey worked. The press was kind. It was more than kind; it was eloquent.

The school authorities were impressed by the quality and variety of the education. The county and city Poor Departments looked benevolently on the work being done for its young citizens and promised some assistance, in spite of the fact that this was a Catholic organization. That assistance was to fluctuate widely through the years, but it never quite disappeared.

Bishop Timon, meanwhile, continued to fight on a different but related front: access for Catholic clergy to public institutions for the poor. Many of the residents of county or privately-run facilities were Catholic. Most were immigrants. In places like the House of Refuge in Rochester and the Protestant Orphan Asylum in Buffalo, priests were still denied freedom to visit, to give religious instruction, or to administer the sacraments to Catholic residents.

Timon was especially distressed about the effect this would have on the children. He encouraged parishes in the diocese to support Catholic orphanages, ordered special collections and set up Orphan Fairs. Not all responded positively to these fund-raisers.

One particularly vocal pastor, Father Daniel Moore, called for systemic change. His letter to a local paper urged

Catholics to pressure the civic authorities for help rather than continuing to hold "these ever-recurring and never-ending fairs." With some drama and venom he wrote:

> I am led to entertain these sentiments...by the contemplation of the odious tyranny to which over 20,000 Catholics in this community are subjected by the bigoted portion of the population in Monroe County. I do not refer to the legalized proselitism [sic] of the Home of Refuge where a few gentlemen are invested with the power of prohibiting the exercise of the Catholic religion to about 200 children. Nor to the House for Idle and Truant Children, wherein every poor little vagrant is imprisoned and the Catholic priest also debarred. Nor to the Friendless Home, where the dying girl is refused the last consolations of religion...I call attention of the Catholics in the city solely to the atrocious conduct of the well-paid gentlemen whom the law invests with the irresponsible authority of Superintendents of the Poor...who forbid me giving instruction to the 80 or 90 Catholic children whom poverty and crime have congregated in that white-washed sepulchre called the Monroe County Almshouse.[8]

This was a battle that John Timon never saw won in his lifetime. It would be 1872 before the Almshouse had a chapel and allowed Catholic services, and 1875 before the House of Refuge permitted a Catholic chaplain for its residents.

Meanwhile, Park House was bursting at the seams. By 1867 there were one hundred fifty boys to be clothed, fed and educated by four Sisters. It was impossible to receive all the applicants. They had to find a larger place.

Early started begging. Three more Sisters were sent from Buffalo to help. Within months they had enough resources to purchase an old building on West Buffalo Street, across from St. Mary's Hospital. St. Mary's Asylum raised $9000 and the state contributed a (token) $1000.

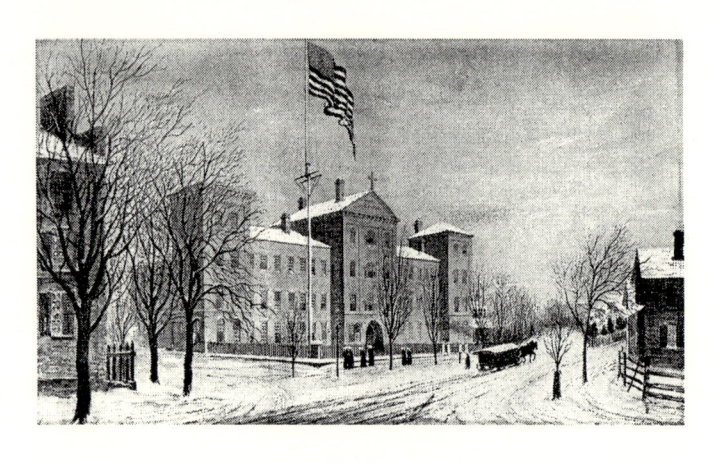

left: Halstead Hall
center: St. Mary's Hospital

Halstead Hall had been built in the early 1830s as a country tavern and inn. During the war it had been used as an overflow residence for wounded soldiers. It was not in the finest shape. The Sisters did what they did best: cleaned, polished, pressed, boiled, painted, hung, fluffed, waxed, smoothed, marked, sewed and moved their boys into a roomier, cleaner, more comfortable new home by year's end.

There was plenty of land around the place - five acres- giving the boys room to run, explore and generally let off steam, a luxury they had not had on South Street. There was even an old quarry nearby that served as a swimming hole after a rain and a hangout when it was dry. The boys' lives were regular and relatively peaceful, a contrast to the violent streets and pounding poverty of the ethnic city neighborhoods or the Almshouse.

People continued to be impressed by the ingenuity and humanity of the young superior. In the first four years St. Mary's had accepted four hundred boys, most of whom stayed a short time, long enough for their families or friends to do what had to be done to provide for them. The one hundred fifty who remained as permanent residents had to be "at home" there, the only home they had.

Sister Stanislaus was well aware of this and had to deal with a delicate balance - providing an environment where the boys would be safe, secure, healthy; where they could grow, be educated, be brought up; where there would be discipline, religious training, "family" traditions. Since the whole set-up was artificial and non-family, this was not easy. It was up to her and the others to create a community, if not a family, among them and to attend to their emotional as well as their physical needs.

The children depended on her; the other Sisters depended on her; the work never ended. She learned young how to protect herself, how to couch her words in formulae and understatement, as later letters would reveal; she learned how to use her femininity both to help and to get what she wanted.

James Early, a magnet of controversy

James Early knew the treasure he had in Sister Stanislaus. He would do anything to make this venture work. His role seemed to be in what is now known as development. Early had influence among the prominent men in the diocese; he was considered Timon's right hand man. The bishop had, in fact, submitted his name as possible bishop for Rochester when the diocese would be divided. Early had many traits to recommend him for this: he was a local man, the bishop's confidant; he was progressive, compassionate, activist; he was young enough to give stability to a new diocese, old enough to have experience as organizer, pastor and administrator. And he knew the clergy.

Later, Bishop McQuaid would blame the serious troubles he had with Early on Early's ambition and his disappointment at not being chosen first bishop of Rochester.

James Early was not universally loved among the Sisters, some of whom thought that his influence with their Superiors had been too strong, and that he used his considerable charm for his own ends. Sister Stanislaus was one of those Superiors.[9]

On April 16, 1867, the same month as the move to Halstead Hall, Bishop John Timon died. Years of trouble and travel had taken their toll; he had been failing visibly for a year or more. He had tried to pave the way for a successor to be left a more governable diocese than Buffalo had become.

The year before, he had promised the congregation at St. Patrick's in Rochester that soon they would have their own diocese, though his petition had not yet been approved by either the American hierarchy or Rome. It was not until January of 1868 that the decision was made to establish a new Rochester diocese and not until March that bishops were appointed: Father Stephen V. Ryan for Buffalo and Father Bernard J. McQuaid for Rochester.

4 THE BEST AND ABLEST OF FRIENDS

In 1868 the Episcopal See of Rochester was created. On the 12th of July the Rev. B.J. McQuaid, founder and for many years President of Seton Hall College, was consecrated Bishop...To the young and struggling community of St. Joseph the Prelate became, in the hands of Providence, the best and ablest of friends, as well as Superior and Father.

Annals, Sisters of St. Joseph of Rochester

Modern psychologists would have a fascinating study in Bernard John McQuaid. At age eight he was orphaned. His mother had died, the victim of disease, when he was three; his father, the victim of violence five years later. Bernard felt rescued from the indifferent, even cruel care of a real-life "wicked stepmother" when a family friend took him to the Sisters of Charity at Manhattan's Roman Catholic Orphan Asylum. The Sisters and other children became his parents, his family, his teachers, his friends, the sum total of his world.

Given the pious atmosphere of that most Catholic of institutions, it is no wonder that the serious young man was off to a seminary when he left the orphanage at fifteen. But he never forgot where he had come from. In years to come he would show his gentlest face to orphans and give them a disproportionate amount of his attention and personal support. And he had seen, in the Sisters of Charity, what women could do.

Bernard McQuaid paid his priestly dues as country curate, pastor, Cathedral rector and diocesan administrator in the diocese of Newark, New Jersey. He founded Seton Hall College, as well as a diocesan community of Sisters of Charity.

McQuaid was a man of many faces. Stern and rigid in appearance, he had a fairly thin skin and could be deeply hurt by unjust charges or personal insults, especially from the clergy. He never quite left the vulnerable orphan boy behind. Determined and single-minded, he himself admitted that the more opposition he received, the more determined he became.[1] He knew how to dig in his heels.

One of the strongest advocates for Catholic education for children, he always regretted that children did not seem to like him. He knew he was fearsome. Not a religious, he lived the evangelical counsels in his own way: spare and simple in his life-style, detached in his dealings with women (and vigilant that his priests be the same), conscious always of the power he possessed and of the obedience it demanded.

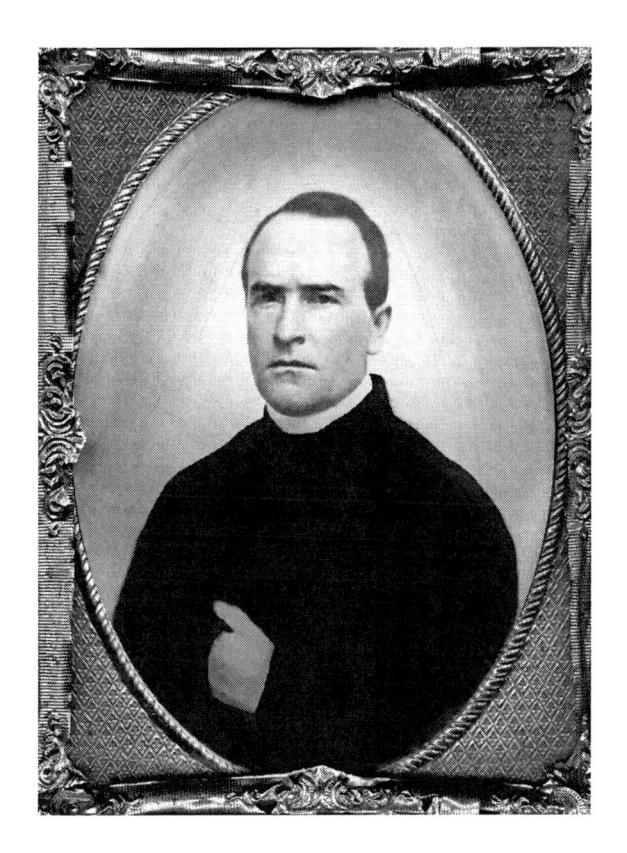

A tintype of Bernard J. McQuaid as a young priest

An eloquent speaker, he could be blunt and curt in social exchanges. He was said to be "more like St. Jerome than St. Augustine."[2] Fiercely loyal to friends, he was a formidable enemy when the friendship was over.

He was a man who got what he wanted. When he came to Rochester, McQuaid had a clear agenda: education for priests and for children. He would do whatever was necessary to achieve both.

By this time James Early was pastor of St. Patrick's, the church destined to become the cathedral. It fell on him, both as Bishop Timon's former Vicar General and as cathedral rector, to welcome and orient the new bishop. He seemed to have brushed jealousy and disappointment aside, graciously assuming his role of second-in-command.

McQuaid himself was homesick. Shortly after his arrival, he wrote to Dr. Michael Corrigan, his successor as president of Seton Hall, "Every now and then my heart feels like sinking within me. No doubt *friends* will be found in time. In one sense, I am surrounded by friends, but they are after all only strangers."[3]

Early's companionship, as well as his knowledge of the churches and the clergy, were invaluable to the new bishop. The two did become friends: Early a trusted ally, McQuaid a respected superior. But, beyond that, friends. Years later, when McQuaid felt that James Early had betrayed him, the bitterness would be as deep as the friendship had been.

McQuaid finds his Sisters

Bishop McQuaid turned at once to the work at hand. Item One on his agenda: free Catholic schools for all Catholic children. He knew that if he were to make his dream of a viable school system work, he would need the labor of women religious. He needed a diocesan Sisterhood, formed specifically to run the schools.

They had to be totally diocesan, not governed by any other jurisdiction, including Rome. They had to be young, flexible, willing to be guided and formed by him, so there would be unity of method and discipline. And they had to have a rule that allowed him freest rein in the ways he could use them in the diocese.

McQuaid made a tentative request to the Sisters of Charity in Emmitsburg Maryland, the order that staffed St. Mary's Hospital and St. Patrick's Orphanage. There were restrictions in their rule against working with boys. They refused.

He inquired of the Sisters of Mercy, who had worked so long in Rochester and Auburn. Restrictions in their rule hindered them, too, and they were under papal jurisdiction as well. He was aware of some ongoing personnel problems in the community that John Timon had worked on. It did not feel like the climate he was looking for.

He needed complete freedom, utter cooperation and obedience. In New Jersey he had been superior of the Charity community he had begun; he wanted the same authority over his diocesan Sisters. The Mercy superior, Mother Mary Camillus, made it clear to McQuaid that she would not be able to hand over the governance of the community to him, as he required.[4] The Sisters of Mercy were off his list. Permanently, as it turned out.

He read the new constitution of the Sisters of St. Joseph that John Timon had fought so hard to get approved. He knew he had found his community. The constitution named the bishop of the diocese as the highest superior: the Sisters were ordered to show him "profound respect, submission and obedience in all things"; he had the power to oversee finances, to correct faults and offenses, to make new regulations as he saw fit, to interpret the constitutions, to assign superiors and Sisters (even to send them to other dioceses, if he wished), to appoint and remove superiors at will.[5]

The bishop, in short, was king of the Sisters of St. Joseph. He would have been a fool to let them go. And Bernard J. McQuaid was no fool.

There were sixteen or so Sisters of St. Joseph working in what became the Rochester diocese: in Canandaigua and St. Mary's Asylum. The bishop gave them a choice: return to Buffalo or stay and form a separate

Rochester community. In the written accounts of this time, it sounds simple. He established a diocesan Sisterhood. Period. It was not simple; it was painful.

Birth pangs of a new community

Asking them to become a new community was asking them to give up their friends, the community they had entered as young girls, their history as religious. It was asking them to leave home as surely as they had left their family homes not so many years before (most were in the community only three or four years); it was leaving them open to even more loss.

It was also an adventure. In America the West was being settled. Young men and women were leaving secure eastern homes and traveling into a vast and unknown frontier. Adventure was in the air.

This would not be a journey into the unknown; it was more a cutting off, a slicing of the umbilical cord. Only three or four returned to Buffalo in the end.[6] Those who stayed could not have known how completely they would become the creation of Bishop Bernard McQuaid.

In Buffalo Mother Magdalen Weber, who John Timon had "borrowed" from Philadelphia, returned home after his death. Bishop Ryan presided over an election and the Buffalo Sisters chose Anastasia Donovan, who had entered with Margaret Leary, as their first elected Superior General.

For Buffalo it was a re-founding. They had lost good friends, a superior they had loved and appreciated, and a strong advocate and patron in Bishop Timon. Anastasia was a kind and simple woman who had been perfectly content at the Dunkirk orphanage, where she had spent most of her religious life. The burden of helping the community recover from its considerable losses and start again fell on her generous but inadequate shoulders. Within two years she would resign, her spirit broken by unwanted responsibility.[7]

For Rochester it was a new creation. Perhaps it was James Early's recommendation; perhaps Bishop McQuaid had had occasion to visit St. Mary's Asylum and had been impressed with the young superior there; perhaps, recalling his own lonely childhood, he had been touched by the progress being made there with the boys. Whatever his reason, Bishop McQuaid saw in Sister Stanislaus the qualities he wanted in the leader of "his" community.

He appointed her as Superior General of the new foundation. Once the decision was made, things happened quickly. The superior in Canandaigua, Sister Elizabeth Wheeler, had returned to Buffalo. The now-Mother Stanislaus sent Sister Ignatius Hanlon to take her place, a decision she would soon regret. St. Mary's Asylum became the motherhouse and novitiate.

It was a struggle. The Sisters had to get used to the facts: They were now to be governed, not by Buffalo, but by one of their own, a peer. Financially they were on their own. They would not be bailed out by Buffalo if, as often happened, they were not paid a salary. The training and education of new members was now up to them.

Those new members included Mother Stanislaus' own younger sisters, Nellie and Bridget. They had been girls of seven and nine when Margaret Leary left home. Most likely they had had minimal contact with her in the eleven years in between, and though they were sisters, they were probably not yet friends. That would come.

Almost immediately the new Bishop of Rochester had to leave. 1869 marked the start of the First Vatican Council, and Bishop McQuaid, a junior prelate, packed up in November 1869 and was gone until the next April. Letters fluttered back and forth. McQuaid had started things and then had left them. One of the things had been the new community he had adopted and promised to lead. The "foundress" was twenty-seven years old; the group was young, small in number, and under his command.

James Early, the new Vicar General, was left in charge of the diocese and of the Sisters of St. Joseph. He and Mother Stanislaus kept the bishop informed (probably better than he ever wished to be informed. The bishops at Vatican I were undoubtedly busy about matters far more serious than the trials of a little New York diocese.)

Fears of scandal

In April 1870 Mother Stanislaus wrote to McQuaid, still in Rome:

I must tell you...that I deeply feel the interest you manifest towards our Community. I hope we may make ourselves worthy of it; with God's help the troubles you anticipate will not occur. If we are circumspect in the reception of Postulants, we can avoid trouble and scandal.[8]

What specific trouble McQuaid had anticipated is not clear, but there would have been reason for his caution. Convents and nuns were the objects of continuing scrutiny and mistrust in the United States. Religious habits, the mystery surrounding their community life, the seeming unnaturalness of the vows, the European manners of most congregations of Sisters had made them objects of ridicule, suspicion and even brutality in the 1840s and '50s. The hatred of foreigners and Catholics had found an easy target in these women.

A plethora of lurid stories had left its mark on the American imagination. Gothic novels pictured young women, imprisoned against their wills, in eerie castle-like convents, helpless victims of sadistic superiors and venal priests; "Escaped nuns," many of whom had never seen the inside of a convent, took to the lecture circuit, spoke to full houses, spinning compelling and imaginative tales of life on the other side of the wall. Pamphlets, tracts and newspaper articles abounded, inventing and repeating incredible exposes of life in the mysterious cloister.

Rochester had seen some of this hate-mongering. In October 1848 two speakers had come to Minerva Hall. "Rev." E. Leahey, an Irishman claiming to be an ex-Trappist (he had been a servant in a Trappist monastery), appeared in a monastic habit to lecture on the "unchristian treatment of females in the confessional, by Popish priests," and "Popish Nunneries." On the same program was Rev. Alessandro Giustiniani, a former Italian priest, a well-known anti-Catholic lecturer, whose topic was: "The United States, being a Province of the Pope, also on Nunneries." Only men were admitted to these lectures. Ladies and young men were prohibited, said an advertisement, "as some awful disclosures will be made."[9]

Twenty years later, Bishop McQuaid was cautious. Even though nuns were no longer openly ridiculed; even though, thanks to the work of the various communities of Sisters in Rochester, in hospital, orphanages, and other social services, their ministry was appreciated by the civic community, their cloistered lifestyle and other-worldliness made them exotic puzzles in a country which prided itself on a spirit of independence and progress. Bigotry dies hard. McQuaid wanted no chance of trouble in this new community. He and his new superior would deal quickly with any problems in the ranks.

Something was wrong (again) in Canandaigua. James Early had been in touch with McQuaid about the superior, Sister Ignatius, who had been acting strangely.

Mother Stanislaus continued, in her letter:

Sister Ignatius is somewhat better and able to be around, she was not able to leave her bed for two months past. Fr. Early told me he had mentioned to you that she had been reading bad books; but I think this is a mistake, the only book she read was a pamphlet left at the door in Canandaigua concerning what was called [indecipherable title]. When she read it, reason forsook her for some time; if she had observed her rule she would not have read it; the transgression brought its own punishment...(but) her mind was impaired before; she is now in a fair way of recovering. She is no trouble whatever to us.[10]

Unfortunately, the title of the troublesome book is impossible to decipher. Could it have been some tract by a proselytizing group in the area? Were there threats or accusations like those so familiar two decades before?

Mother Stanislaus coolly blames what seems clearly a breakdown of some kind on a small infraction of the Rule. The practice of blaming God when faced with inexplicable mishaps or trials has always been an easy "out," but in this case it didn't have much credibility.

Ignatius had entered the community seven years before, from Peterborough, Canada. She must have shown maturity and leadership to have been named superior of the Canandaigua mission. Mother Stanislaus' assertion that "her mind was impaired before" seems odd. There is evidence that Sister Ignatius had difficulties with the pastor, Father English. But, then, so did Mother Stanislaus, as she complained to Bishop McQuaid:

I found the Sisters had more orphans in Canandaigua than they can well support, we have been trying to diminish the number. The proceeds of the Orphan Fair amounted to about $1000, this is not enough to support and clothe twenty-five children and seven Sisters; the Sisters have not received a Selery [sic] for teaching since Father English came there; he thinks the Fair enough.[11]

Mother Stanislaus appointed her friend Sister Xavier Delahunty as superior in Canandaigua, and this seemed to mollify Father English. James Early saw the situation differently. A month later he reported to

McQuaid: "Father English is much pleased at the Sister who has charge of the Community in Canandaigua. Everything goes on remarkably well and he is doing everything to assist the Sisters and encourage the schools."[12]

A good politician, Early must have known that the remark about encouraging schools would please McQuaid. Paying the Sisters was evidently not his concern either. In fact, when he was himself pastor in Canandaigua, he did not even allow the fair to be held; the Sisters and orphans existed on the money from music lessons, the academy, and whatever they could get form the state Poor Fund. This battle for just wages--even subsistence wages-- would be an ongoing one.[13]

The community *Annals* handles Ignatius delicately, merely saying that "unfortunately, she did not persevere."[14] Actually, she asked to transfer to a cloistered community, where she stayed only a short time before joining another group. Fifteen years later she would write to Bishop McQuaid, begging him to allow her to return to Rochester, since Mother Stanislaus was no longer in power there. Ignatius' memory of her time in Canandaigua is quite different from Stanislaus' words about her:

> You know, dear Bishop, that I have never complained of any unjust or unkind treatment received at the hands of Mother Stanislaus, nor is it my intention to do so now, after keeping silent for so long a time...I don't know what reasons Mother Stanislaus gave you at the time for my desiring to make the change but I am certain of this: that she did not treat me in a candid, straightforward manner...I was very young and inexperienced and she took advantage of both my youth and ignorance to carry out her own ends...this afterwards I saw, though at the time I was too simple to understand fully her workings.[15]

As a superior, Ignatius would have been responsible for helping to evaluate new members and, evidently, she had crossed Mother Stanislaus on one very personal evaluation:

> I don't know of any reason for her unkind conduct towards me except that on one occasion I opposed, as far as I could, the reception of one of her sisters into the Community. This I did from a conscientious motive, not being able to discern in the Aspirant any sign of a Religious Vocation...her manner of acting towards me was changed from that time forward.[16]

In the same letter Ignatius hints at some financial difficulties from that time which she had "thought it virtue to keep silent about." Whether this refers to Father English's refusal to pay the Sisters or some accusation against the Reverend Mother is not clear and will never be known. One thing is certain: she wanted to come back and thought the coast was clear:

> I have been in [indecipherable] for the past twelve years and I have felt like a sojourner in a strange land, longing to get back to my own state and diocese. I knew this was not possible, so long as Mother Stanislaus was at the head of the Community.[17]

Ignatius had a certain flair for the dramatic. She describes her life as "Egyptian bondage."[18]

Bernard McQuaid refused her request. He never even brought it up to the community's council for their consideration.

Sister Ignatius was not the only one from this time to request a return to the Rochester community. Not long after his installation as bishop, he had been warned by a lay Sister at the Canandaigua orphanage, Sister Augustine Humphrey, that James Early was not to be trusted. She had been summarily sent away to Dunkirk, in the Buffalo diocese, dismissed from the new community.

McQuaid had to be able to trust his Vicar General. He depended on his counsel and experience. He did not know who this woman was or what her motives might be for trying to discredit James Early.

A letter from the past

Who was this Sister Augustine? I found her letter quite by accident in the Rochester Diocesan Archives. It was mixed up with a number of receipts for Excelsior Farm, one of McQuaid's short-lived projects of the '70s.

Blue onionskin paper, thin as air mail, the writing nearly illegible because it is written in layers, pages five, six and seven crossing over pages one, two and three, written sideways over the other writing. "Crossing" I'm told, was common practice in those days. It saved paper.

I wonder if McQuaid ever read it at all. I'm sure no one has, since.

It took weeks of painstaking "translation," but as I pieced together word by word, phrase by bitter phrase, the story of a lonely and shattered spirit emerged from the tortured script.

Free and easy she is with spelling and grammar. Her run-on sentences would make even Dickens wince. Some words are hopelessly illegible and my translation is full of _____'s, like names and places in old Victorian novels.

"I am the Sister," she begins, "You ordered to be sent out of the diocese for informing you of the [indecipherable] of J. Early."

But this is not about James Early. This is about the sadness of a spirituality and a system that put some people over others, in God's name, of the sadness of caste and privilege and hierarchy.

50

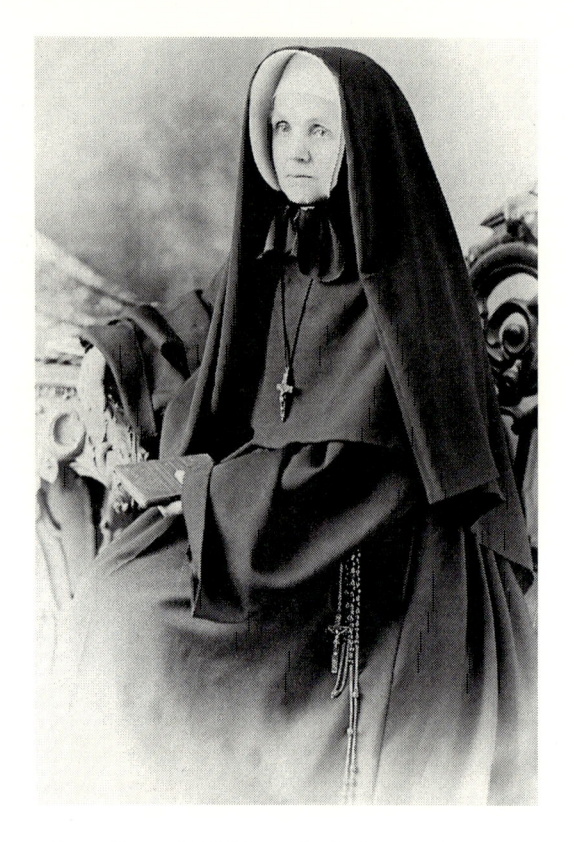

Sister Patrick Walsh in the habit of a lay sister

Among the Sisters there were still two distinct classes. The choir Sisters were educated and did the public ministries. They were the teachers, the administrators. The lay Sisters, often poorly or un-educated, did the menial work. They were a servant class, distinguished even by their habit, which was different from that of the choir Sisters. In a world where rank mattered, they ranked lowest. This was a carryover from the community's European roots, always troublesome in American branches, but not yet abolished.

Her letter continued:

"I was the first candidate in Buffalo, bringing with me one hundred dollars hard earned from doing plain sewing for a family while I was waiting for an opportunity to enter a religious order."

She was twenty-five, an English orphan girl named Ann Mary Humphrey. A convert, a woman who felt a call to something. Sister Stanislaus was seventeen, then, and much was made of her:

"And the young Sisters from Canandaigua were made superiors in the missions and those who entered the Buffalo Asylum, the Bishop made them lay Sisters as he wanted them to work for the orphans."

There is a tightness in her tone, as though she were squeezing understanding out of the memory, as though the writing were itself catharsis for the pain of being passed over.

"And at the same time they were receiving subjects without any means in Canandaigua and educating them for quire[sic] Sisters...I never asked for anything more than what I got until now..."

Bishop Timon had promised her that in time she would receive the choir habit. Then Mother Agnes Spencer left; the community was in turmoil; the bishop forgot his promise.

"I am broken down from fifteen years hard and heavy work, from Dunkirk to Canandaigua, doing the baking and washing for the Sisters and the orphans...but the hardest cross for me is to be despised and disrespected because for the love of God and my neighbor I have taken the lowest place...religion exalted them and degraded and lowered me."

The handwriting is quick and sharp. The letter is an open floodgate:

52

"My religions are more respectable than any superiors or Sisters were in Buffalo or Rochester, half of them were hired gurls [sic] and could not bring one hundred dollars, but they got the quire [sic] habit...my brother considers me a disgrace to him to be under the feet of everyone..."

Her brother owns a flour mill. He is ashamed of her:

"But being a Protestant, he doesn't know anything about humility."

Her parents had had money, but her father squandered it and both had died young...

"..leaving a large family. So my brothers and Sisters were raised by our aunts and uncles and all received a plain education and the boys a trade and all of them are in business for themselves and my Sisters are just as respectable."

She came to America when her brother was established. She roomed with a Catholic girl and became the only Catholic in an otherwise "respectable" family.

"And since then I have never looked back. God's grace has been sufficient for me, to do his will which had always been my happiness."

Her simplicity is poignant. Happiness? When has she been happy? The portrait she draws of her life reveals drudgery, not ministry; humiliation, not humility; being used, not being useful. Wearied by work, she spits her bitter envy to the page. She is an innocent; she believes their assessment of her - their superiority and her lowliness. Until now.

"The superior here will give me the veil with your order as I cannot return without honor, it is only justice, I am only asking for what I should have got first. I was able to fulfill all the duties required by my

holy rule except teaching and I have never used one hour of time to study, but there is plenty of young Sisters to teach what they have learned at the expense of the community..."

Finally she claims her own talents:

"I can do plain and fancy sewing work, a great many of those cannot do it but I am not particular where it is fine or corse [sic], ruff [sic] or smooth..."

But she knows she must gain the attention of the bishop. Her words grow mean and bitter; they tumble out without organization. She speaks of Father Early as though he were some Svengali who "gained the heart of both Superiors and got inside God and the community and everybody else."

He is a "Crowned Devil," she says. He left debts in Canandaigua, she says. He is no friend of the Sisters or the orphans at St. Mary's she says. He likes his glass of punch too much, she says. He hurries through his spiritual exercises and is no priest, she says. He is too fond of Mother Stanislaus, she says. This is a sad letter. A reader sifts out the silt, keeps the sand.

Bishop McQuaid did not let her return. He would hear no criticism of his Vicar General. Buffalo has no further record of Sister Augustine, only a handwritten note on her profession document: "1868, Belongs to Rochester,"

Rochester mentions her nowhere at all.

5   THE OLD BALANCING ACT

> *(sisters)... were the Catholic serfs, having fewer rights and fewer options than priests, brothers or lay people. Bishops possessed the ultimate authority and frequently sought to interfere in the internal affairs of the community. Some pastors treated them worse than hired help...Obviously all bishops and pastors did not act in this manner, but those who did were so numerous that this aspect of American Catholic history would constitute a book in itself.*
>
> Jay P. Dolan, The American Catholic Experience

We seem to measure time in decades. Though they are not as clean, clear, and delineated as we would like them, they are convenient.

Some snaps from the 1870s in Rochester: Unions. Strikes. Violence. Susan B. Anthony has the effrontery to register to vote. She is arrested. Small pox, meningitis, tuberculosis. Death wore a young face. Immigrants fear that freed slaves could take their jobs; a depression carves a new gap between the rich and the poor. Telephone lines go up. George Eastman starts a little company he calls Kodak, nonsense syllables that sound to him like the click of a camera. The Great Snow Blockade: the railroad stopped, the city stopped.

An odd event took place in Rochester in 1872 that suggests that our moral compass was not as true as the city fathers would have us believe. Accounts refer to it as the "Howard Riots." An old history relates the story:

A Negro named Howard was accused of assaulting a white girl.

Was Howard his first name or his last? It doesn't seem to matter. He's just Howard.

On his arrest he was placed in the jail, which then stood on the island between Exchange Street and the river...an angry mob gathered in the vicinity intent on lynching the culprit.

We always thought we were civilized up North. This city, especially, was cultured, liberal-minded, compassionate. We had been so morally superior during the war. But not above a little lynching.

The 54th Regiment was called out to defend the jail...the rioters provoked the soldiers, who fired a volley, killing two men and wounding five others...

Kent State? Selma? Frightened young soldiers; riot police nervously fingering a trigger? Who's to blame? It's an old question.

A secret session of the court was held at night. Howard, whose face had been whitened with chalk, was smuggled into court and induced to plead guilty, whereupon he was sentenced to the State prison in Auburn for twenty years. That night he was taken to Honeoye Falls in a carriage and on the next day was lodged in the prison at Auburn, where, if we mistake not, he was murdered by a fellow convict.[1]

Some accounts say he was pushed from a window; some say he was stabbed. In any case, the city bore the guilt. Good people saw the dark side of themselves. The city was not yet forty years old and had already lost its innocence.

The Catholic Church (that subculture) and women religious (that subculture of the subculture) found their way through the seventies on a parallel track, straying to intersect only on occasion. Their snapshots are different: row upon row of sleeping orphan boys; somber young blackrobed Sisters in faculty picture, fingering crosses or rosaries, glancing away from the camera's eye; churches rising in all phases of construction: brick, stone, stained glass, carved wood.; immigrant workers, smiling; schools, children with folded hands, straight backs, pressed, combed, beribboned.

Their innocence was intact for now.

Mother Hieronymo recalled

After he returned from Rome, Bernard McQuaid heard that Sister of Charity Mother Hieronymo O'Brien (Rochester's Florence Nightingale, founder of St. Mary's Hospital, respected by civic leaders, a legend to soldiers, loved by the poor, bearing the heavy burden of being popularly canonized while she was still alive) had been transferred to New Orleans.

The city fathers were incensed. They demanded her return. Their demands were ignored. McQuaid moved quickly. He well knew that St. Mary's Hospital, which accepted patients without distinction of race, religion or ability to pay, was the firmest symbol of good will towards

Catholics in Rochester. And Mother Hieronymo, in the minds of the people, *was* St. Mary's.

In October of 1870 McQuaid wrote to Father Burlando, the Vincentian who was the Sisters' superior, asking him to withdraw the Sisters of Charity from St. Patrick's Asylum. He had plans, the bishop said, to move it to a larger location and to give its management to the Sisters of St. Joseph. Burlando, thinking this was a retaliation for taking Mother Hieronymo away, offered to reinstate her if his Sisters could stay at St. Patrick's.

The suggestion of some sort of bargain infuriated McQuaid even more. His decision stood, no matter what Burlando did about Mother Hieronymo. He accused the Vincentian of insensitivity to the church in Rochester, of endangering the future of St. Mary's, of alienating Catholics and Protestants alike, of causing scandal in his refusal to listen to the pleas of citizens who demanded Mother Hieronymo's return. Burlando stood his ground and Mother Hieronymo went to New Orleans as ordered.

The Sisters of Charity took annual, rather than perpetual, vows. When her annual vow expired, Mother Hieronymo left the order and returned east. McQuaid had an idea. He urged her to join the Sisters of St. Joseph. Then she could be a religious and stay in Rochester for the rest of her life.

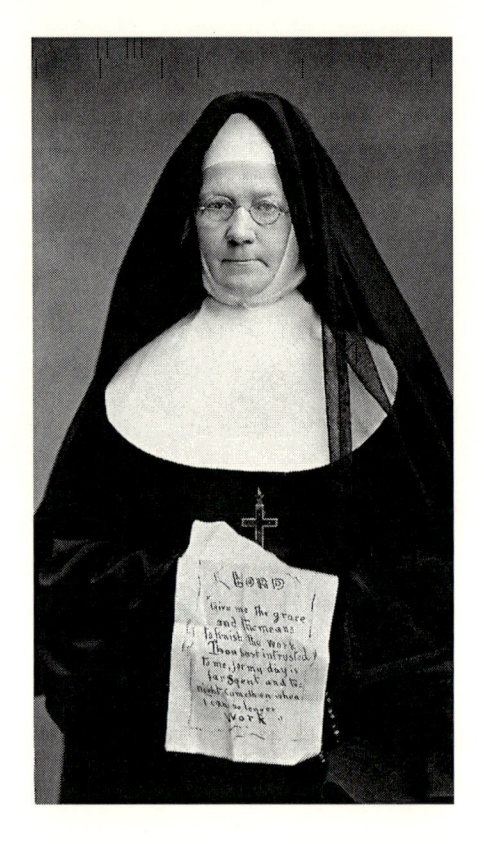

At Bishop McQuaid's urging, Mother Hieronymo O'Brien transferred to the Sisters of St. Joseph but her heart remained with the Sisters of Charity.

    As for St. Patrick's Asylum, the bishop made good his threat to remove the Sisters there and replace them with "his" community. The Sisters of Charity had been at St. Patrick's for twenty-seven years. McQuaid had accused Father Burlando of insensitivity to the people. It would seem he was blind to his own.

St. Patrick's Girls' Home: caught in the controversy

It had been the Sisters of Charity, not the diocese, who had kept St. Patrick's afloat for almost three decades. Old account books record money earned from "industry of Sisters," "industry of inmates," "Sisters' teaching," "fair proceeds," and a curious one-time-only notation: "collected from Protestants 12/30/65."[2] It had been the Sisters of Charity whose devotion to the orphans had endeared them to the people of Rochester and had earned them the respect of city and state charity officials. And it was these Sisters whom the children knew and trusted. One could not simply pull them out, insert new bodies, and continue as though nothing had happened.

As with many bishops of the time, McQuaid acted as though women religious were commodities to be used interchangeably and at will. Personal talents were sometimes considered; personal feelings were not. In November of 1870 he inserted six Sisters of St. Joseph at St. Patrick's: three would run the select school, two would care for a hundred thirty orphan girls and one would teach the eighty children in the free school. The six left Halstead Hall on a cool November morning. The driver hoisted their bags to the twelve-seat State Street horsecar that would take them to St. Patrick's. It was not a long ride.

The orphanage was a boxy, three-story brick building behind the new cathedral. Forbidding, institutional and utilitarian. Not much energy had gone into its aesthetics.

Inside, things were different. One hundred thirty girls, toddlers to teenagers, came to meet their new Sisters. Nervousness on both sides. The older girls wore their good black dresses; they had dressed the little ones in their good white muslin. The place smelled of wax and had an antiseptic "convent" look. That, at least, was familiar.

The children took them on a tour: a formal parlor for visitors, a music room, two large classrooms (one with a fine melodeon for singing class); upstairs, a quiet little chapel ornately furnished in the taste of the time.

Across the hall was the clothes room, filled with numbered shelves and wardrobes: dresses, skirts and shirtwaists on one side; hats, high button shoes and hair ribbons on the other. Each child had a number to match her belongings. All the clothes were handmade. Most touching of all was the dormitory for the "baby girls," rows and rows of tiny beds, the bedding boot-camp neat, where preschool children slept.[3]

The children took them through sewing rooms, classrooms, playrooms, dining rooms and, finally, the large community room which would be the Sisters' only private place. On a large secretary desk lay the Sisters of Charity's account book. It had one final entry: *Nov. 1, 1870 . Sisters left. Cash on hand: $1,000.00*[4]

There were layers of emotion here to be sorted out. The children, already orphaned, had lost the only mother-figures they had known. The adjustment would be hard. Their relatives and the Catholic community who had supported the asylum for so long were angry that the Sisters had been forced to leave. Rumors were fierce about the whos, the whys, and the hows in the switch.

The work itself would be exhausting. Sister Francis Joseph (Mother Stanislaus' sister, Bridget) was assigned to organize and run the free school. She had worn the habit less than a year; she had no experience whatever. Later she recalled those days.

During the first year we were subjected to the insults of the people, as we were supposed to have been the cause of the sending away of the Sisters of Charity, to whom the people were devotedly attached. God gave us the strength in those days to go through many trials and difficulties.[5]

Eventually people's attitudes towards them changed, but the harshness of the beginning of that mission would remain with them a long time.

Sister Evangelist Haggerty attributed their eventual success there to the notion that they had only been obeying the bishop, and that God blessed obedience.[6] It probably had more to do with the fact that the next year Sister Hieronymo O'Brien entered the Sisters of St. Joseph and took over the management of St. Patrick's Asylum. She was a link between the old and the new. People trusted her. Everybody relaxed.

The motherhouse and novitiate moved for a time to St. Patrick's, to alleviate the space problems at the boys' home. Already the community had grown to twenty-eight, more than doubling their number in two years. Mother Stanislaus knew they needed a place of their own.

McQuaid saw it, too, and explored several sites with her. They decided on a large home and acreage on the corner of Jay and Frank Streets, the property of Major John Williams, a retired army man. It was only two blocks from the bishop's residence. He would be a frequent, even daily, visitor when he was in town--to the schools, to the convent, to the children's home. Though the name on the deed read "Mary Stanislaus Leary, Superioress," there was no mistaking who was the real superior of this order.

They called the house Nazareth. Almost immediately they closed the select school at St. Patrick's, brought the faculty and girls to the Jay Street building, and called it Nazareth Academy.

The free school at St. Patrick's Cathedral remained as the first in McQuaid's new parochial system. He would have no more "poor schools." Each parish would support its own school; Catholic education would be free to all Catholic children.

Life in the orphanage

Halstead Hall was cramped and crumbling. The trustees of St. Mary's Asylum drafted a petition to the New York State Legislature, asking for support for a dormitory wing and repairs to the building, which they claimed as "about to tumble down." Their appeal was simple, even poignant:

...the building...is out of repair, rickety, cold and entirely unfit for the proper accommodation and comfort of the little children within its walls. It is too small; the little fellows are packed away into every available corner, having no well-ventilated dormitories, no play room in which to exercise in the wet and wintry weather.[7]

They asked the legislature for $20,000, appealing to their sense of justice and responsibility for the children of the state. From the records it is not clear whether they succeeded in convincing them that a religious-sponsored institution should be supported by state funds, another perennial question.

The money came from somewhere, because by 1872 they had collected enough to build a central building on to Halstead Hall. And each month's receipts showed an entry from public funds.

The accommodations, while more spacious, were far from homey. Dormitories slept fifty boys at once; the Sisters shared rooms in two and threes, and one Sister slept in each dormitory in case a child needed help or comfort in the night.

The Sisters in both orphanages were rarely away from the children, never away from responsibility; some of them were hardly more than girls themselves. They had a strong work ethic that kept them cooking, making beds, doing laundry, mending clothes, combing hair, fixing ribbons, matching socks, teaching lessons, monitoring study, reading stories, giving baths, supervising playtimes, buying provisions, putting on fairs, disciplining errants, figuring finances, while trying to maintain some semblance of a religious life among themselves.

But it was not the discomforts, fatigue or everyday frustrations that bothered them most. They learned to live with the old balancing act: strictness vs. affection, individuality vs. conformity, training vs. education, accessibility vs. a need for privacy. They worried about what would happen to the children when they were too old to remain in the safe cocoon of the orphanage. Sister Hieronymo and Bishop McQuaid shared this concern and had some creative answers.

The Home of Industry and Excelsior Farm: creative answers to "aging out"

Sister Hieronymo set aside a section of St. Patrick's as a Home of Industry for girls. Her program was two-pronged: further education and practical training for older orphan girls and a safe home for young working women. Within a year they had outgrown St. Patrick's and she purchased two small houses on Edinburgh Street, in the affluent "ruffled shirt" district of the city.

Hieronymo had a knack for funding her projects. The residents and Sisters supported themselves from the room and board of the working girls and from their own labor. They advertised in the Rochester newspapers as specialists in tailoring, slipper and shoe making, made-to-order ladies' and men's clothing; they appealed to churches to give them orders for vestments, altar linens and church decorations; they opened a laundry service. By the time a young woman left the Home of Industry she had employment or the skills to obtain it.

Bishop McQuaid saw the value of the Home of Industry and wanted a similar project for the boys at St. Mary's. He purchased a sixty-five acre farm on Charlotte Boulevard in 1873, called up the services of the Sisters of St. Joseph, and began Excelsior Farm Industrial School. Here older orphan boys would live and learn to grow vegetables, tend orchards and vineyards, work in the canning factory and winery. They would work for their room and board and receive useful training but no salary. Their "contributed services" would keep the place going.

The Sisters took care of the house, taught in the little school, and presided over the canning factory. Imagine it: thirty or so teenage boys, working at assembly-line speed, processing and canning, in silence.

Excelsior Farm was praised by local merchants who purchased their quality canned goods and by the State Board of Charities as well. The bishop took a very personal interest in the work, often working alongside the boys in fields and factory. If mere enthusiasm could keep a project alive, this one would have flourished. But it lasted only six years. Not enough boys stayed on to staff it. It was a good idea that failed.

6 ORDINARY TIME

> *The 'good nuns' may have been the subject of jokes in male-chauvinist rectories and their outlandish costumes no doubt produced nightmares in many a schoolchild...they were often unappreciated and taken for granted by Catholics. Yet the Sisters were absolutely essential for Catholic schools. The American bishops had solemnly decreed...that every Catholic child should go to a Catholic school, but without the Sisters they would have been powerless to execute the decree. The Sisters worked for next to nothing and their dedication could not have been purchased with money.*
>
> Edward Kantowicz, "Schools and Sisters" *Corporation Sole*

By the mid-1870s the years of dramatic change and painful choices had given way to ordinary time. The community annals reveal a group (and a superior) who had settled in, who had found a focus: Catholic schools. Each year the Sisters began a school or two, dotted all over the diocese.[1] It became clear that they were the "chosen," that they were inextricably bound to this diocese, to this bishop, to this work. The loyalty on both sides seemed unshakable. But privilege was a two-edged sword. Eventually the Sisters paid the price.

The other women's congregations in the diocese McQuaid ignored without apology. With reason the Sisters of Mercy felt this most deeply and for decades would feel the results of his neglect. McQuaid would not allow a community to receive candidates unless there was a specific work for them to do. Only three schools were in the care of the Sisters of Mercy during McQuaid's long tenure.[2] The Sisters of St. Joseph had the most schools, the most jobs and, consequently, the most candidates.

The School Sisters of Notre Dame were well established and needed in the German-speaking schools and they, like the Sisters of Charity, were governed by far-away headquarters. Rochester was mission territory to them, not home. They did not feel the sting that the Sisters of Mercy felt when McQuaid restricted Mercy candidates or repeatedly sent the Vicar General to preside in his stead at their reception and profession ceremonies. He was not a subtle man.

There is no evidence that either Mother Stanislaus or her community was aware of any hostility or resentment on the part of the unfavored congregations in those early days. Later they would know of it. In fact, a competitive spirit grew between the St. Joseph and Mercy communities in Rochester, an uneasiness that would last a hundred years or more.

Such interpersonal problems would not have touched Bernard McQuaid at all, though his cool favoritism was clearly their source. He seemed to care only that his community was flourishing; that meant a growing work force to staff his schools.

Bernard McQuaid gave the Sisters of St. Joseph his full attention. He became their chaplain, spiritual director, master teacher, benefactor, and vocation recruiter. He might as well have written SSJ after his name. Nazareth was so close to the Cathedral that he could easily drop in at any time. And drop in he did. He delighted in interrupting a study hour to quiz the novices or a classroom to instruct the children or (more likely) to admonish a teacher. A young Sister Amelia Hennessey recalled that he came to school every day:

>...the least disorder or want of method on the part of the Sister presiding in a school room were noted and corrected with unerring promptitude. A paper on the floor, a mark on the wall or furniture was noted and measures taken to prevent the repetition of so grave neglect on the part of the young teacher.[3]

Every Saturday he said Mass at Nazareth and gave a conference. Often the talk included mention of faults and infractions he had noticed in a classroom during the week and advice on how to improve not only their spiritual lives but their teaching methods as well. McQuaid's spirituality and theories of religious life informed theirs. Frequent themes ran through his instructions:

Women can do (almost) anything. They are the best teachers because they are "soft."
There is no work nobler than Catholic education.
Sisters should have as little as possible to do with priests.
The more the suffering, the greater the merit.
The basis of true religious life is "work and obey."

His was a no-nonsense approach to God: work hard; say your prayers; do as you're told; don't whine; be loyal. "All your efforts," he told them, "should be business-like."[4]

Freedom, mystery and subservience

Every year new candidates came, steered to the community by the bishop. The numbers were not unique. It was happening all over the country. The 1870s and '80s were years of astounding growth in women's religious congregations in the United States.[5]

Why? A nun's life was rigorous. It involved long hours of prayer and physical labor, the sacrifice of sexual love, motherhood and family life, voluntary poverty, and the submission of will (and even intellect) to a Superior. What was the attraction? In spite of privations, religious life offered women a career, a certain freedom of movement that wives and mothers were denied; it presented more choices to single women who often ended up working in factories or domestic service. Sisters had an opportunity to live in a secure community, to forge bonds of friendship with other women, to test out their talents. Even though their lives were described and circumscribed by rules, even though they were set apart by cloister and habit, there was in their lives a paradoxical freedom to initiate programs, to be visible in the public arena.

There was, too, a mystique about a nun's life that had always fascinated people. There was an appealing romanticism in the religious habit, the secrecy of the closed cloister, the notion of denying human love to be a Bride of Christ, of leaving all things for God as a sort of human sacrifice.

Popular Catholic devotions in the nineteenth century could only have confirmed a young woman's attraction to such a life. Most Catholics left theology to the priests. The devotional life of the ordinary Catholic was based on the senses more than the intellect, on the concrete rather than the abstract. Faith was expressed in a multitude of prayers, often written in ornate and flowery prose; in devotions to various parts of the body of Christ (blood, wounds, face, hands, feet, head, heart, side) each an earthy, understandable symbol of Christ's relationship to us; in reverent displays of sacramentals (scapulars, holy water, medals, rosaries). In this religious climate, Jesus was real and reachable, prayer was experiential, and suffering was redemptive. It is easy to see how a life of asceticism, shrouded in mystery, layered with the romanticism of a "mystical marriage" would appeal to a young woman of limited options. Curiously, choosing a life of submission brought them a certain power, a chance to have some influence in the society and in the Church; leaving the world offered opportunities to travel it more widely than they might have if they had married; renouncing marriage gave them a freedom to meet men as peers, at least in their work. In the Catholic community, at least, women religious had some status and respect; in the wider community they were gaining respect (even if it were sometimes grudging) because of their work in hospitals and orphanages.

For some, religious life offered adventure in the mission territories; for others it meant the opportunity to found and run schools, hospitals, social service agencies. Sisters became knowledgeable in finances, corporate structures and operations, even construction. They were often educated younger and more thoroughly than their Sisters "in the world."

And if they seemed subservient to the men who ran the Church, that did not seem to deter them. They did not question their place (the same place as other women in society). Instead, they learned how to work within (and around) that place. They did not feel the need to join the women's movement that was bubbling up all around them. In fact, they seem to have taken no notice of it at all.

In Rochester, while Susan B. Anthony was giving speeches, gathering supporters, getting publicity from her daring attempt to register as a voter, Sister Hieronymo O'Brien was quietly founding the Home of Industry. Her contemporary, Jenny Marsh Parker, wrote:

The truth finds illustration in what has been attained for the advancement of women by the quiet innovations, women who never spoke from a suffrage platform, and are shy of suffrage conventions, but who believe that the world belonged to those who take it...We have had no women aspirants for legal honors, nor has a single one permitted Reverend to be written before her name, unless it be the truly reverend Mother Hieronymo, who may bear the title as fittingly as any one upon whom it was ever bestowed-- the founder of St. Mary's Hospital and the present venerable head and inspiration the Home of Industry.[6]

At the same time, Mother Stanislaus Leary was learning how to be the president of a growing corporation, Nazareth Convent and Academy. From the Jay Street headquarters, she assigned personnel to eleven new missions, directed major construction projects, oversaw the financial affairs of the community, planned for the education of the members, saw to the physical, emotional and spiritual needs of the Sisters. And dealt with the bishop. Not many thirty-year-old women had that sort of responsibility in the 1870s.

As for the Sisters, there is an upbeat tone in the accounts of that time. They were busy - even overstretched- but there was a general *esprit de corps* among them, a feeling that they were creating something together. Some may have called it mere conformity. There was definitely a mold into which a young woman was cast if she wanted to be a Sister of St. Joseph. A certain image and spirituality were carefully cultivated, even in the earliest years.

The original French influence was apparent. Formal prayers were emotional, with emphasis on sinfulness, unworthiness, sorrow, self-effacement. Early community prayer books abound with litanies, examinations of conscience (page upon page of possible ways to sin!), devotional prayers to be said during the Mass (in counterpoint to the priest's prayers).

Pious practices, such as kissing the floor, kneeling

to a superior, Chapter of Faults, asking for penances for minor infractions, praying with the arms extended *("les bras en croix"*), and use of the discipline (a small metal scourge that a religious used on herself to remind her of the sufferings of Christ) were European monastic carryovers that the Sisters adopted without much question. It is curious that it was almost a century before the Rochester Sisters of St. Joseph abandoned these oddly masochistic practices, while in their work they continued to be modern and progressive.

Externals were carefully orchestrated. In public the Sisters lowered their veils and covered their hands; they did not look gentlemen in the eye nor shake their hands; they did not run or "walk with precipitation"; their habits were identical, even to the width of the hems in their linens and veils and the length of their sleeves; they did not draw attention to themselves. Their Customs Book told them that "their passions should by mortification be tranquil and subdued, and from their exterior everything childish and trifling should be banished. The Sisters should stifle the very first irregular movements of the passions."[7]

These, of course, were ideals. It is to the credit of all religious who survived this sort of training that there was always a gap between the real and someone's notion of the ideal. The same book and some quaint, funny advice as well, such as these hospitality hints:

Sisters who visit other houses should be saluted with the kiss of peace and receive polite attention. It would not be polite to inquire into their business or to ask such questions as 'With whom did you come?' or 'When are you going home?'[8]

The operative virtue in those days seems to have been submission. The community annalists make much of it. They mention two Sisters who seemed promising, even brilliant, but who could not conform.

One, Sister St. John Baptist from New York City, who had been referred to the community by Mother Stanislaus' old friend Baptista Hanson, is described as "brilliant and generous" but lacking the necessary humility:

> Sr. St. John Baptist was endowed with many gifts by nature and wherever she taught her boys liked her and to this day speak in her praise. But with those gifts nature had enjoined a dominant disposition and an impulsive character which in subsequent history proved the cause of calamity to her.[9]

Another, Sister Sienna Quinn, was "a very brilliant Irish lady...a graduate of the Dominican convent of Cabra near Dublin...an accomplished musician but...never made for the obedience and submission demanded of a religious."[10]

At the Second Plenary Council of Baltimore, the American bishops had made it clear that the "good religious" was one who was separated from the world. There had even been a short-lived schema called "De Clausura," proposed at the First Vatican Council, which would impose cloister in some form on all women with simple vows. It did not fly, however; other more pressing matters (such as defining infallibility) took precedence so the proposal was not addressed. The idea would be picked up again around the turn of the twentieth century, when universal norms began to be drawn up for religious congregations. But that was years away.

So the Sisters themselves learned to deal with the tensions between the requirements of religious life and the demands of their ministries. It was an old question (one that has yet to be resolved). With these Sisters, it became a matter of life and death.

A matter of life and death

The Rochester Sisters of St. Joseph were young, many of them in their teens and early twenties. They were thrown into a rigorous regime of study, teaching, housework and religious exercises. Some seemed exhausted; many, their resistance low, became ill. By 1877 eight young Sisters had died, three of them still novices. The situation was serious, the losses heartbreaking.[11]

Mother Stanislaus, deeply grieved, knew she had to do something. Clearly the young Sisters needed a break, some fresh air, some respite.

Sister Amelia Hennessey, herself a teenager in those sad days, remembers it this way:

> Many, in fact nearly all of our Sisters were barely out of their teens and the building up of robust constitutions was the lookout for the Sisters then. Rev. Mother Stanislaus, in her truly maternal spirit, inspired or helped to inspire the Bishop with an interest more than ordinary in this matter so important for the future of the Catholic schools of our diocese.[12]

This account typically underplays the terrible human toll, the loss of young friends, the grief of the families and the community, twisting the tragedy around to be merely a matter of needing healthy workers for the school system. In some ways, these generous youngsters seemed to be regarded as cogs in a machine.

Hemlock days: controlled relaxation

Bishop McQuaid owned a large home and farm on Hemlock Lake, where he loved spending his time off and entertaining guests. He offered to lease it to the Sisters for a summer getaway and to build a small house on the property for himself. Mother Stanislaus (though she went through all the motions of protesting that oh, no, it was too big a sacrifice; oh, no, the new house would be too small for him; oh, no it was too extravagant for them) accepted his offer. It seemed to be a good arrangement for all of them.

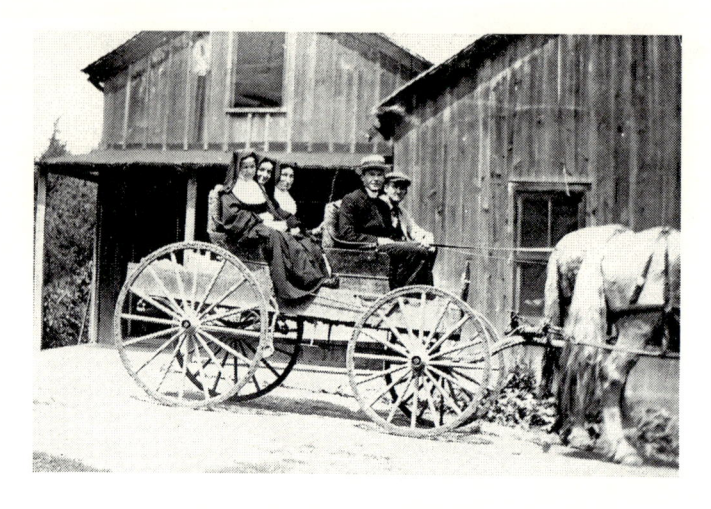

The Sisters enjoy a horse and cart ride at Hemlock Lake

The Sisters who went loved Hemlock. It was just what the doctor ordered. They rested, picnicked, rowed on the lake, soaked up the sun. But even their vacation time was formational.

The bishop was often there at the same time as they and spent a good deal of time getting to know each one. He invited speakers on pedagogy, theology, and spirituality to give short courses to the Sisters.

If they felt suffocated by his attention, no one wrote about it. But their lives were surely not their own, and it must have been frustrating for their Reverend Mother to claim her own authority with them. She was, in those days, absolutely cooperative with McQuaid. Whenever he requested Sisters for a new mission, she found them and found the means to support them. Her letters to him are childlike and submissive, ending always with the standard "Your obedient child" and there is no reason to think that it was tongue-in-cheek.

There was obviously a mutual respect, even a friendship of sorts, between them, though she could not have yet seen herself as his peer, and McQuaid was singularly cautious in his dealings with women. Later correspondence between them reveals a new confidence she finds in herself, and ability to respond to him as an equal. But for now she remained his "obedient child."

Mother Stanislaus was able to find support and friendship from others during these first years: from her sisters Nellie and Bridget, from her friend Mother Baptista Hanson, to whom she always turned in trouble. Baptista had served a term as Mother Superior in Brooklyn; she could well appreciate the burdens that her young friend was carrying.

Stanislaus kept in contact with others who were leading new communities: Mothers Mary Anne Burke in Buffalo, Agnes Spencer in Erie, Marie Sidonie Rossle in Jacksonville. They were all feeling their way, and relied on each other.

Early and McQuaid: a bitter parting

Mother Stanislaus took James Early's support for granted. They remained trustees of St. Mary's Asylum and continued to work for that institution they had founded together over a decade before.

But James Early was in trouble. He and McQuaid had lived together at the Cathedral for eight years. Now there was an evident erosion of their originally congenial relationship. Something--or perhaps a number of things--

had happened.[13] For one thing, St. Patrick's Cathedral labored under a heavy debt. Constant improvements, added to the ordinary expenses of running a large church, had left the parish with an $82,000 debt. Early had lent the parish some money of his own, but there never was enough. At the very least, the bishop questioned the rector's management.

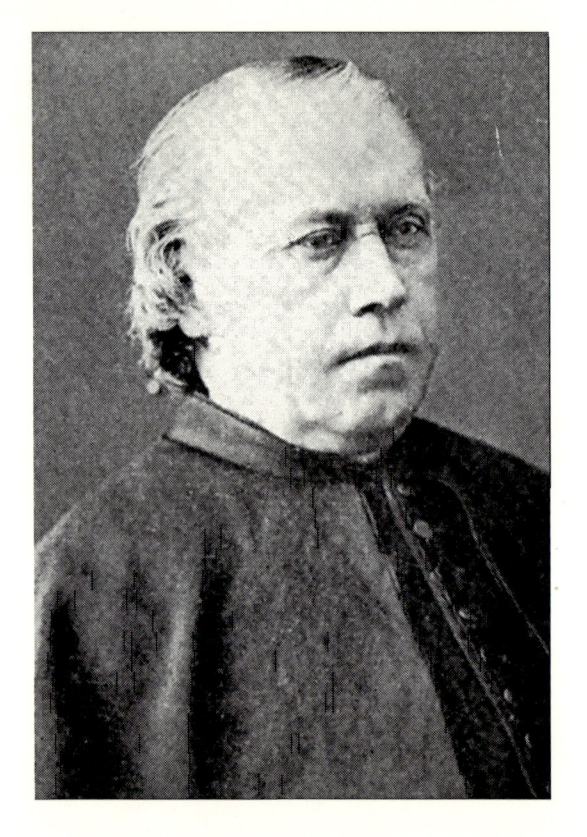

Father James Early

In 1876 James Early requested and received a transfer back to the Buffalo Diocese and, after he left, began a legal suit against the Rochester Diocese to collect interest on loans he had given St. Patrick's. McQuaid, angry and hurt by this unexpected blow, wrote scorching letters about Early to his Episcopal friends and to Bishop Ryan in Buffalo. He accused Early of causing scandal that (he predicted) would be far-reaching; he spoke of Early's "diabolical hatred" that would give way to "gross vilification and abuse." He appealed to Bishop Ryan to step in and order Early to withdraw his lawsuit. Ryan refused to get involved in what he saw as a personal disagreement between McQuaid and Early.[14]

There were hints of the unrest even in the records of St. Mary's Asylum. From the beginning, the trustees had kept careful records of their meetings, decisions and financial dealings. Father Early and Sister Stanislaus had been president and secretary/treasurer, respectively, of the Board of St. Mary's, which they had founded together. Their personal influence on the organization was strong and controlling. As early as 1871 Bishop McQuaid replaced Early as president. There are no more minutes or treasurer's reports recorded until April, 1876, when James Early is listed as absent from the meeting. By then he was also "absent" from the diocese, and another priest was quickly appointed to take his place.[15]

Perhaps it was in these years that Mother Stanislaus began to see Bishop McQuaid in a new light. She could not have been happy about the feud that had arisen between two men she considered her friends; to support one would mean disloyalty to the other.

The young priest whom McQuaid had chosen to succeed James Early as Vicar General and Cathedral rector, had been carefully selected. James O'Hare had grown up on Frank Street, in St. Patrick's neighborhood, attending St. Patrick's Academy with the Christian Brothers. A quiet intellectual, O'Hare was an astute businessman. He had built the church, rectory and school at St. Bridget's and had kept the place in the black. When McQuaid appointed him to St. Patrick's, O'Hare begged him (in tears, on his knees) to find someone else.

Among other things, he did not think he would be accepted in his own home parish. James O'Hare was James Early's opposite: serious and thoughtful to Early's good-natured bluster; delicate and ascetic to Early's husky energy and pragmatism; steadily intellectual to Early's erratic activism.

Above all, he was unconditionally loyal. McQuaid would take no more chances. He would groom this young man for greater things. James O'Hare would be like a son to him, perhaps a successor.

But the new rector was not naive. He knew that James Early's departure (under mysterious circumstances) had not been easily accepted by many of the Cathedral parishioners. Early had made devoted friends in every parish he had led. People were simply attracted to him ("Bewitched," Sister Augustine Humphrey would have said). O'Hare did the best he could to help the parish heal, but he spent most of his energies reducing the debt and supporting his bishop.

He was cool in his relationship to the Sisters of St. Joseph, as cool as James Early had been hearty. His name is rarely mentioned in the written records of those days, even though he had reason to have had frequent contact with the Sisters in his offices as pastor, neighbor, trustee of both orphanages and Vicar General.

And while James O'Hare kept his distance, the bishop continued to be a part of the daily life of the community, now free from Early's influence.

7 DAYS OF THE MIRACLES

On May 16, Rev. Leiter S.J. from Canisius College gave a retreat for the Academy girls. He was remarkable for his gift of tears...Julia Holmes had hemorrhages from the stomach and wonderful visions in consequence.

Annals, Sisters of St. Joseph of Rochester

Schools were the focus. Teaching, Bishop McQuaid kept saying, was the noblest Christian work. "There is not a charity in all this country," he told them, "hospitals, asylums, refuges of any sort which for far-reaching, widespread and lasting charity can for one moment be compared with our Parochial Schools."[1] Everything had to be done to insure the success of the Catholic schools, to make them comparable in secular studies with the public schools.

When Cathedral and Immaculate Conception schools opened on 1871, neither building was completed. Inexperienced teachers struggled to keep discipline while carpenters hammered away and the children maneuvered their way around ladders and hardware and painting paraphernalia. In spite of a bad start, within a few months there were eight hundred children at Cathedral and five hundred at Immaculate Conception.

The concept of free parish schools spread quickly, as McQuaid exhorted, encouraged, even bullied his priests and people into making Catholic education their first parish priority. And not only in Rochester. In Brockport, Avon, Webster, Auburn, Geneva, and Seneca Falls rural and small town parishes built their schools, sometimes even before they built their permanent churches.

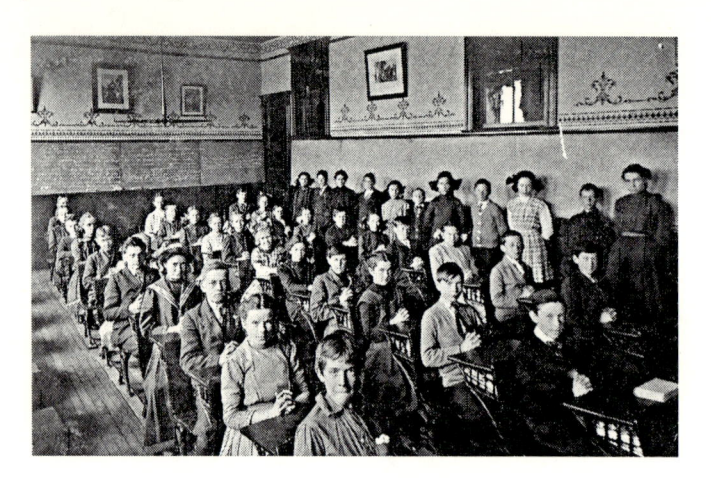

A Catholic school classroom

Some beginnings were difficult. Auburn's St. Alphonsus Church tried three times to establish a school. In 1870 Sisters Catherine Mullen and Tecla Reichert opened a little school in the town's Academy of Music. Sister Tecla had only worn the habit six months, and was charged with teaching German to a class of eighty students. The boys took full advantage of her youth; she couldn't handle them at all. Sister Catherine wryly recalled:

During the first week of school, a Fair for the benefit of St. Mary's Church [Auburn] was being held in the same building--the Academy of Music, and, imagine if you can how pleasant this was for us. The boys would repeatedly ask to leave the room, only to go to the Fair, the noise and confusion of which made all school-keeping all but impossible.[2]

One morning, only a month after the school opened, the Sisters returned from lunch to find a note on the door saying that they could no longer use the building. They closed for a week and reopened in a forbidding-looking building near the railroad tracks. The first floor was a hardware store, the second a tobacco factory. The school was on the third. Behind the building was a tannery. The odors of the tannery and tobacco factory mingled noxiously; the street car and railroad cars roared past them at regular intervals. A bad situation became impossible. They lost heart.

Mother Stanislaus called the two home at the end of the year. She would not subject her Sisters to unreasonable hardships. They were certainly ready to make sacrifices for the schools, but she drew the line when it seemed that the churches were unwilling to give them basic necessities for their ministry. The bishop could not have been pleased with her decision.

St. Alphonsus Church opened another school two years later, this time without Sisters. It closed after six years. The Sisters returned in 1887, when Mother Stanislaus was no longer in charge, and that time it worked.

In April, 1876, the school in Dansville, New York was all ready to be opened, when a smallpox epidemic broke out just south of the little town. A quarantine was ordered. Highways leading to the town were closed, and travelers required to bathe in carbolic acid before they entered Dansville. When the quarantine was lifted that summer, the town had a double celebration: the start of St. Mary's School and the centennial of the Declaration of

Independence.

Mother Stanislaus took five Sisters to Geneva in September of that year, to begin a school at St. Francis de Sales. The Sisters arrived in time for Sunday Mass, and as soon as they saw the number of children, Mother Stanislaus sent a message to the motherhouse, asking the Mistress of Novices, Sister Adelaide, to pack her things and join them. They opened the school the next week with three hundred fifty children. Even with six Sisters, the teacher-pupil ratio was nearly sixty to one.

Most Genevans had not seen nuns before and, though they were hospitable, they made no secret of their curiosity. Sister Matilda Flaherty, one of the first group, remembered: "When we entered the church for Mass every head was turned to survey us, and when we came out it seemed as if every inhabitant of the town was there assembled."[3]

Two weeks after their arrival, the bishop came to see how they were faring. He asked a young priest who was in charge in the pastor's absence if the Sisters had everything they needed. The priest, flustered, relied, "No, Bishop, but I am going to get them some holy pictures next week." Sister Aloysia bent her head to McQuaid's and said, "Bishop, we have no flour in the house."[4]

Each year the Academy and the parochial schools held public exhibitions to show off their skills and their learning. The children regaled their guests with recitations, musical programs, debates, drama and poetry. The Academy girls loved performing. Mother Stanislaus hired Mary Anne Noah, a retired professional actress, to work with the students in drama and elocution. Mrs. Noah was the first of several teachers at the Academy hired especially for training in the arts.[5]

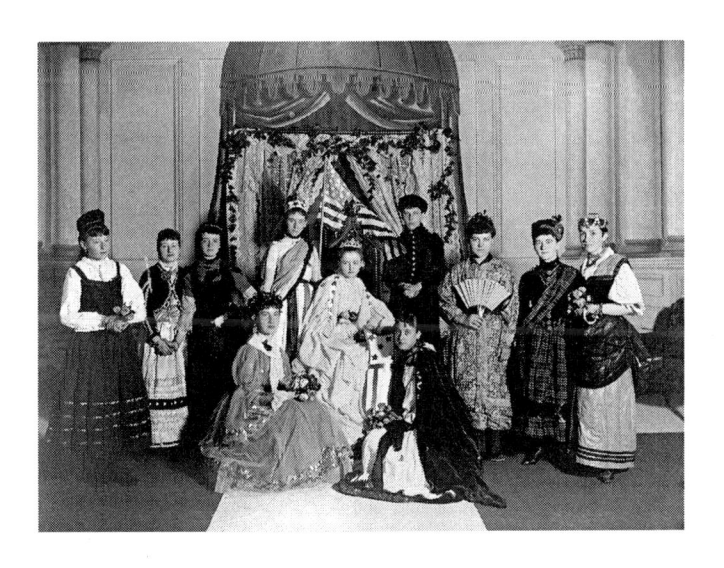

Students at Nazareth Academy present a play with an international theme

But the arts, fulfilling as they might be, were not enough to keep the schools competitive. By 1878 the exhibitions had become more serious, more academic. Cathedral school held public examinations. For four grueling days parents, priests, friends and educators came to observe the children, who were questioned on stage, first by the priests, then by anyone else in the audience. At Nazareth Academy the girls "analyzed sentences, parsed words, spelled down, worked problems, etc. to the intense interest of those present."[6] Hardly exciting by today's standards, but it paid off.

Soon the Catholic schoolchildren were passing state Regents examinations and getting notice from state authorities. But it wasn't enough. Though the Sisters had extraordinary dedication and the best will in the world, they needed education. They needed to learn how to teach.

Luckily, they had connections. The diocesan chancellor was Monsignor Hippolyte DeRegge. He had come early to Buffalo as a Belgian missionary. McQuaid had taken him to Rome as his theologian during Vatican Council and the two had toured Europe in search of art, books and vocations for the diocese. A gentleman ("by birth, nobility and character" as an obituary described him),[7] DeRegge was a sought-after preacher, a charming host, a brilliant conversationalist, an unassuming friend of the poor, a stern Catholic. His chivalrous manner made McQuaid's gruffness all the more apparent.

DeRegge had been instrumental in sponsoring a young Belgian teacher, Rosalie Frison, as a postulant with the Sisters of St. Joseph. Mlle. Frison had been trained at *L'Ecole Normale de St. Andre* in Bruges, one of the best teacher training schools in Europe. McQuaid and Mother Stanislaus decided that this would be the place to send some of their best minds who, in turn, would begin a Normal School in Rochester.

Rosalie Frison, now Sister Berchmans, had received the habit with a brilliant young woman, Sister Seraphine O'Kane. Seraphine and even younger Sister deSales Feeley were chosen to be the pioneers.

McQuaid was planning on an extended European trip in the autumn of 1878 and had hoped that they would go with him as far as Belgium.[8] He would enjoy getting them settled, giving them advice, showing them off like a proud father. For some reason, they couldn't leave for a few more months, so McQuaid reluctantly sailed without them.

The following January Sisters Seraphine and deSales boarded the Cunard steamer *Celtic* in New York. Once in deep water, the ship lost its propeller and, according to Seraphine, the officers and crew looked to the two nuns to pray for a miracle, since nothing short of that would save them. They prayed. The ship was saved.[9]

But they were used to miracles in those days. In 1875 the *West End Journal* printed the story of the "miraculous cure" of Sister Mary Chrysostom at St. Mary's, Auburn. According to Dr. Loughlin, the pastor, Chrysostom had been dying. She had been anointed, had been "in her agony" several times. The doctors were waiting for the end:

> On the evening of June 30th, at a moment when her condition was as bad, if not worse, than at any former period of her illness, it was suggested that the water of Lourdes should be applied to the sufferer. The Sisters consented to do so and recited nine Hail Marys before and after making the application. Scarcely was the last Hail Mary concluded than Sister Chrysostom exclaimed, "I am well." and asked permission to rise. She actually leaped from the bed and joined with the Sisters in the singing of the "Te Deum," though her tongue had been so thick and inflamed in the morning that she could not receive Communion. Shortly after this Dr. Guerin...entered the room and seeing the change that had been wrought...exclaimed "No human power could have effected this!" Sister attended Mass the next morning and has been perfectly well ever since.[10]

They were blessed with an uncluttered faith. They expected miracles and miracles happened. No one was surprised when the ship was saved. Sisters Seraphine and deSales reached Belgium without further incident and began their rather rigorous studies at St. Andre's. They were homesick. Because of the cost they would not be returning home for holidays or vacations, but would remain overseas until they had finished their course.

Back home things were far from dull. Nazareth was expanding all the time. Mother Stanislaus had directed that the building be raised one story, topped with a handsome mansard roof. She had purchased the property that abutted theirs, so there was a bigger yard and room to build a brick stable. She had told McQuaid of her plans for the expansion of the motherhouse and, sensing in him a strong opposition to the project, she waited until he went to Rome before initiating more improvements! She couldn't have known that he had plans of his own.

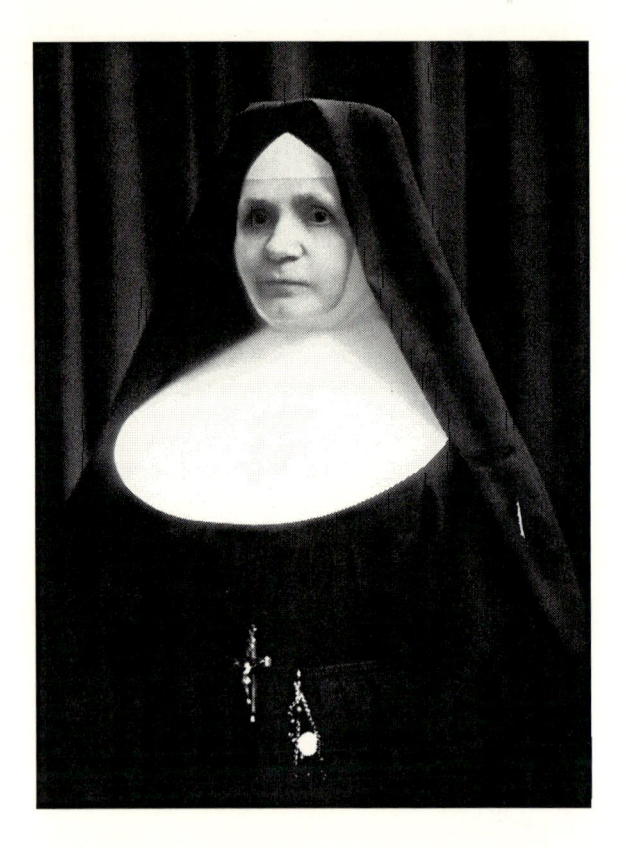

Sister Berchmans Frison was a teacher in Belgium before entering the Sisters of St. Joseph. As writer of the Annals, her words and interpretations color what we know of this time.

Sister Berchmans was appointed as Mistress of Novices (though she was barely out of the novitiate herself); Sister Agnes Hines, a quiet, artistic young woman who had held that office became Mother Stanislaus' assistant and, at least at first, her friend.

If Sister Agnes was shy in those days, Mother Stanislaus had found her own stride. She was not as easily controlled; she seemed more aware than ever of her responsibilities to those trusted to her care and authority. She was especially concerned about the health of the Sisters. The deaths of all those young people had affected her deeply.

So far she had been able to assign Sisters whenever they were requested by the bishop or pastors, but her Sisters were stretched. Many worked too hard, mistaking pure endurance for zeal. They still were often not paid or paid below-subsistence wages. The bishop kept telling them to cut back, pull together, save, sacrifice. He would not be pleased, she knew, when he saw the improvements she had made on the motherhouse while he was away.

Then the unexpected happened. At the end of January, Bishop McQuaid, still in Rome, received a frantic telegram from an acquaintance from Rochester who was traveling in Naples. With him was a physician who was extremely ill with a deadly typhoid malaria. McQuaid went immediately to Naples to see what he could do. The doctor died quickly and McQuaid used his influence to help with the necessary and complicated arrangements.

On the train back to Rome, he himself fell dangerously ill. He had contracted the disease and literally fought for his life for several weeks. He wrote his friend Bishop Corrigan that, "No one in Rome except one physician believed it was possible that a man of fifty-five years could possibly live through such a sickness."[11]

The Sisters prepared the school children for his homecoming. (Only those who have worked with little children on a performance can fully appreciate what that meant.) Mother Stanislaus went down to Hemlock to get his house ready.

If B.J. McQuaid had any doubts about how his people felt about him, they must have been dispelled on April 27, 1879. He stepped from the train at Erie Station, was whisked into a carriage drawn by four white horses, driven down streets lined with thousands of cheering people, and taken to St. Patrick's Cathedral. Inside hung huge banners, Episcopal red-and-white:

VIVAT BERNARDUS
JURIS DEFENSORI
PATRI ORPHANORUM

Music, speeches, cheers. The affection was sincere, the relief in having him safely home, obvious. He was deeply moved.[12]

The Sisters and children got their chance to greet him not long afterwards. First, the Academy girls: little girls strewed flowers in his path as he entered the new reception hall (one of the surprise projects done while he was away. He surely had mixed emotions in seeing *that*!); then each age group stated a welcome in a long, formal program.

But the reception that touched him most was, predictably, at St. Patrick's Orphanage. Seventy small girls ("merry girls of silvery voice") sang a greeting song; then little Minnie Thompson stepped forward, handed him a bouquet, and gave a welcome speech. McQuaid's usual gruff demeanor melted:

The Bishop was deeply moved at the affecting address and heartfelt gift and he acknowledged his gratitude in a very feeling and eloquent manner. He said that the little bunch of flowers he held in his hand was dearer to him than he could tell...because it was the unsolicited offering of innocent little children for whom our Loving Savior has such a predilection. He told them that he knew, "when he lay on his bed of sickness well nigh unto death, that his dear little orphans in the city of his home were not unmindful of their father at the sweet hour of prayer."[13]

He loved being called "Father of Orphans." He was back. Full steam. It was as if he were never gone.

While he was away, in March of 1879, Mother Stanislaus had received a letter from a Mrs. DeVaney, the rectory housekeeper in Dansville, telling her of Sister Angela Keenan's sickness and desire to come home to Rochester. Mrs. DeVaney had nursed Angela through a winter of illness. Angela had sometimes been "blind with pain," she said, and had told her that she would like to go home to the motherhouse to die. Angela would not ask for herself; undoubtedly she thought it virtue to suffer in silence. Mrs. DeVaney spoke up for her.[14]

The talk of imminent death was, it turns out, premature. Sister Angela Keenan died in 1937, aged 85. But Mrs. DeVaney's letter reveals a warm affection between them. Such a relationship would not have set well with the bishop, who was even then in the midst of battle with the Dansville pastor, Father Henry Egler: insubordination, scandalous language and behavior, questionable relationship with his widowed housekeeper. McQuaid had fingered her as an "evil influence" and "at the bottom of his (Egler's) troubles."[15]

The kind and utterly simple woman who wrote to Mother Stanislaus is quite different from the Eve/Jezebel of McQuaid's judgment. He would not have appreciated his Sisters' being friendly with her. But he must have noticed that the superior was not as malleable as she once was.

Mother Stanislaus was never known for her erudition. In fact, she is usually described as "childlike," "simple," "amiable," "liberal," "attractive." The facts of those days reveal someone who had reached a new point of firmness (if not toughness) in claiming her own authority, someone with growing business savvy, someone who would no longer be managed, someone who had an intuitive sense about people, someone who was a natural administrator.

She had learned from James Early how to use her contacts with the well-to-do to get advice and resources for new projects; from McQuaid himself she learned how to hold on with determination to what she felt was right. This was not the same person who had snubbed Sister Ignatius Hanlon for questioning her sister's vocation, or who had been unquestioning in handing over the governance of the community to the new bishop. What she lacked in formal education seems to have been more than compensated by natural talent.

The bishop still had the ultimate power, however, and he was personally involved in personnel problems and decisions. And he was approachable.

There was, of course, no access to a telephone. The first Rochester exchange was established in 1879. It would have been long after that that the convent would have had a receiver and even then its use would have been strictly restricted. So notes were run back and forth from Nazareth to the bishop's residence (a stone's throw) at a sometimes rapid rate. The notes that have survived are an interesting study. Some are mundane, routine requests for an interview or an apology for some minor infraction; some are frantic pleas for reinstatement or understanding. Almost without exception they are letters written to a father-figure, not a distant judge. In spite of normal conventions and formalities of nineteenth century letter writing, these Sisters seem to have felt free to approach McQuaid personally:

"Dear Rev. Bishop, do not read this with that cold frown

you had on yesterday; it chilled me like ice." wrote one Sister.

"Please answer this. I feel dreadful." pleaded another

"I sent so often to the house this morning and last evening, but you were out each time. I will stay here at the Asylum till I hear from you." stated a third, confident that he would reply.

"I appeal to you as a father in my present trial," cried another[16]

    Mother Stanislaus acknowledged the bishop's position as Father Superior even as she claimed more and more her own authority. She was proud of the Jay Street house and enjoyed entertaining Sisters from other foundations. Guests came and went. Mother Mary Anne Burke came from Buffalo, Mother Agnes Spencer from Erie.

    Mother Baptista Hanson came to visit in October. McQuaid did not like her. He thought she had too much influence on her old friend Mother Stanislaus; he thought that she undermined authority.[17] Within three years his anger and frustration with their friendship would erupt dramatically, but in 1879 he seemed to endure her presence quietly.

    Instead of a direct attack, he warned the Sisters about frivolous visits. He did not approve of their traveling about, wasting time and money. He called their attention time and again to the directives in their rule about travel. He had similar admonitions for his priests. In a letter to Bishop Corrigan he gave high praise to some new priests he had appointed who "believe in Catholic schools, pay debts and stay at home."[18] He himself continued to travel frequently on extended European trips and visits to friends in New Jersey and the South. Apparently he saw no irony in this.

The seventies came to an end without fanfare, but as the new decade began, the seeds of unrest, planted deep, started to stir and break open.

8   WHOLEHEARTED, UNQUERYING CHILDREN

> *What fervent, whole-hearted, unquerying children they were-- from 5 A.M. to 9 P.M. studying and working, with fully five hours in the chapel...practicing rigorous self-denial...and withal as merry as children on a holiday!*
>
> Katherine Conway

    Several unrelated events occurred early in 1880, setting the mood for the difficult years that followed. Toward the end of February, Nellie Byrnes, one of the Academy high school boarders, became very ill. It was tuberculosis. Mother Stanislaus sent for Nellie's parents and on March 1, Mrs. Byrnes came to take her home to Lima. Nellie knew that she was going home to die.

    A few days later they had another shock. Mrs. Catherine Jobes was a formidable woman. She had come with Bishop McQuaid from Newark and had been his cook, housekeeper and, above all, doorkeeper for twelve years. She was something of a Cerberus: one did not get past her easily. Priests and people alike were afraid of her. But McQuaid knew her worth. She was unquestioningly loyal, utterly devoted to him. And her abrasive manner was a good match to his own gruffness.

    On March 10 Mrs. Jobes was caught in a fire. She

was deeply burned and near death when she was rescued. There was no point in taking her all the way to St. Mary's Hospital, so they gently carried her the short distance to St. Patrick's Asylum, where the Sisters could tend her. McQuaid was in shock. He fussed about her. He visited her every hour, all evening and into the dark night. She died at 4:00 A.M. One of the Sisters heard him cry out, with uncharacteristic emotion: "Oh Catherine, must I stand here and see you die?"[1]

He grieved a long time for Mrs. Jobes. She had been a link to the past; and she had known him as few in Rochester had.

McQuaid was still in fresh mourning for his housekeeper when Mother Stanislaus became dangerously ill. Her illness was, as usual, unspecified but it must have been severe. The Buffalo *Catholic Times* contained this note:

Reverend Mother Stanislaus, the respected Superioress of the Sisters of St. Joseph in Rochester, was seriously ill last week. We are pleased to be able to say that the worthy lady is now convalescing, for her death would prove an incalculable loss to religion in this part of the vineyard.[2]

Sister Agnes Hines wrote to Sisters Seraphine and deSales in Belgium:

I know it will grieve you to hear that our dear Reverend Mother has been and is yet very ill...Today she appears a little better and the physician has pronounced her out of danger. She will not however be able to get home for at least a week.[3]

Sister Agnes must have had to pick up some of the administrative responsibilities while Mother Stanislaus was sick, giving her some experience that would be needed sooner than anyone could have guessed.

During the first week of May, Nellie Byrnes died,

putting sad closure on the grief that hung over the Jay Street house. Sister Agnes sewed a shroud for her. A group of Sisters and classmates traveled to Lima for her funeral. In the community annals there is a chilly passage about this sad event. Sister Berchmans, with a coldness shocking to modern ears, remarks that Nellie "was very desirous of being a religious, but as she was her father's favorite child, he had not the courage to give her up, so God took her to Himself."[4]

One of the widely-held misconceptions in the Church before the Second Vatican Council was that religious life was a "higher calling," and that standing in the way of a religious vocation was direct defiance of God's will. Sister Berchmans' fearful image of an avenging, jealous God was not uncommon. Even so, her conclusion, that Mr. Byrnes' attachment to his favorite daughter gave God no other choice than to "take her to Himself," is worthy of a shudder or two.

At the end of the school term the teachers at Nazareth and Cathedral School went down to Hemlock for a long vacation. It had been a hard year. They thoroughly enjoyed their time at the lake, but something happened on the way back home that must have made them feel jinxed. Sister Berchmans recalled that trip in detail:

On the afternoon of departure, we had to cross the lake in boats. On the opposite shore a carryall was waiting to take us to Rochester. It was about 4 P.M. when we started. The horses seemed even then to be tired, and we were at one time obliged to walk part of the way, since the poor animals were hardly able to draw the load. To make matters worse, the driver lost his way. Finally, about half-past nine in the night, we reached the neighborhood of Mt. Hope Cemetery. It was very dark. All at once horses, driver and seventeen Sisters were thrown headlong down over a steep bank at the roadside. Impossible to describe the confusion that prevailed. Cries, groans, aspirations were heard.

One Sister's shoulder was dislocated; another's cheekbone put out of joint; a third complained of a broken nose, etc. The whole party was more or less bruised, but none, thank God, was fatally injured. How glad we were to reach home about midnight. When, on the following day we went to Holy Communion, the priest, noticing so many disfigured faces, inquired if the Sisters had been fighting.[5]

    Tuberculosis claimed another victim in September. Sister Mary Joseph Fives was one of those bright, natural teachers everybody wanted to have. She had been made superior and principal at St. Francis deSales school in Geneva and suffered from tuberculosis for over a year, going in and out of remission, regaining her energy and then falling sick again. They had hardly begun the fall term when she died.

    The funeral was in Geneva, and the Sisters from the missions, Seneca Falls, Canandaigua, Auburn and Brockport, joined her Sisters and friends at St. Francis. After the service, six young men, former students, carried her casket to the train station in procession, followed by all the mourners from the church. They watched as Mother Stanislaus and Mary Joseph's own mother boarded the train to take her home to Rochester.

    Nazareth Academy, though still small, was beginning to gain a reputation. It was going beyond the ordinary "convent school" curriculum and using the resources in the Rochester community. The girls visited local industries and the University of Rochester (which must have irritated the bishop, who had made it clear that he thought the university to be a Godless institution and dangerous for young Catholics, especially women); they frequented cultural centers; museums, galleries and concert halls, to expand on the arts education they were receiving at school. Parents interested in a liberal education for their daughters were beginning to show interest in Nazareth.

    And Nazareth was about to have a new, exotic,

peculiar, slightly bizarre addition to their arts faculty.

Alice Seymour: stirring up the pot

In mid-December of 1880, the portress at the motherhouse answered a knock. A fortyish woman, face shielded from the bitter cold by a long hooded cloak, extended a perfectly-manicured hand holding a card that read: *"Honorable Alice Seymour, mistress of English to the Archducal Family of Austria."* The young Sister brought her in, seated her in a parlor and hurried to get Reverend Mother.

When Mother Stanislaus greeted her guest, Mrs. Seymour said that she had just come from the bishop's house. He had referred her to the Sisters. She had returned, she said, from a long tenure as governess to the children of the Austrian archduke. She was a recent convert to Catholicism. She needed a rest. Could she remain with them at the convent for a time while she recouped her strength? (She held the popular misconception that convents were places of rest!)

Mother Stanislaus evidently had her doubts about Honorable Alice Seymour. In spite of the fact that the bishop had sent her to them (and that could easily have been because he had no idea what to do with her), Mother Stanislaus was not about to let her stay without requiring something in return. She hired her to teach the Sisters music and elocution in return for her room and board. She could live in the convent with them. As her strength returned, she could join the faculty at the Academy as well. Mrs. Noah was still there and might welcome another laywoman on the faculty.

Alice Seymour accepted. She would last six months. It was unfortunate that someone as unfamiliar with religious life and so unrealistic in her expectations would have chosen that particular year to become acquainted with Sisters. There was something unnerving about Alice Seymour. As a difficult time unfolded at Nazareth, her presence added an extra measure of concern.

First sign of trouble

By January of 1881 the scene was set. On January 17 Mother Stanislaus received the first blow. She brought McQuaid a letter sent by Father O'Hare forbidding her to have anything further to do with St. Mary's Asylum. She thought the bishop would support her. When she realized that he would not, she lost her temper. Later that day she sent off a note to him:

Right Reverend Bishop,
Please to send me Father O'Hare's letter. I hope you will pardon me for giving way to my feelings in your presence this morning. The truth is, I have so much to contend with of late and so little encouragement or sympathy from where I might expect it, that I am very nervous. I will try with God's grace to overcome myself in future and bear wrongs patiently.
Most respectfully,
Your obedient Child in Xt.
M. Stanislaus[6]

McQuaid's reply is not extant, but he obviously asked her about some unpaid debt, probably a loan St. Mary's had made to Nazareth Convent when she was treasurer.[7] Three days later she wrote:

I here send...an explanation of the debt of $1900. I hope after an investigation of the matter you will find it correct. If I have manifested displeasure at Fr. O'Hare's arrangements, I feel I had good and sufficient reasons. I founded St. Mary's Orphan Asylum in this city under many difficulties, and have managed its affairs for over 16 years and under the circumstances, I receive such a letter, from which I was given to understand I would not have anything more to do with that

Institution, not even a voice in its management, I would be more than human if I did not feel it. However, I will relinquish my interest in its affairs, and I promise you I will not interfere with Father O'Hare's arrangements. I know...it is not your doings, I have expected this change, I meant no disrespect to you for such is not in my heart. I bear towards you...the most profound esteem and veneration. You are my Superior, and to whom could I go in my trials and difficulties if not to you?
I hope you will correct and punish my faults when you notice them. I will always try to obey your orders in the spirit of faith.
I am...with profound respect and the highest esteem,
Your most obedient child[8]
M. Stanislaus

 Even then she trusted in the bishop's good will toward her; she placed the blame squarely on the insensitivity of Father O'Hare. She could no longer get a loan from St. Mary's. They would have to find other ways of raising money. As president of St. Mary's Board, O'Hare was entirely within his rights to question large loans. Her problem lay, not in the fact of his questioning, but in the high handed and punitive method he used with her.
 On St. Patrick's Day Alice Seymour gave a benefit concert for Nazareth Convent. Records show it was a "financial success." Dance was added to the offerings at Nazareth Academy. This innovation was not totally accepted by some on the faculty. Not only was this questionable activity being taught to their own, but Miss Burke, the instructor, had opened it to "outsiders" as well. As Sister Berchmans, always the lady, remarked, "Uncalled-for comments were made on the subject by unreflecting persons."[9]
 Mother Stanislaus seemed impervious to criticism about it; she was determined that the Academy be saturated with the arts and open to the outside world. Alice Seymour gradually settled into the community and seemed to be revered, especially among the youngest, most

impressionable of the Sisters, and others who were awed by her European experience.

Lay women at Nazareth: Alice and Kate

Alice Seymour was not the first lay woman to have lived with the Sisters at Nazareth. In 1870 eighteen-year-old Katherine Conway wanted to be a journalist. She started a small monthly paper called *The West End Journal and Orphan's Advocate.* Its original purpose had been public relations. It featured articles about St. Patrick's and St. Mary's Asylums; it publicized their needs and progress, and thanked individual benefactors for donations; it reprinted pious "Catholic" stories and gave editorial comments on topics of Catholic interest. Gradually the *Journal* included parish activities, school news, priests' assignments and the bishop's schedule. It became, in fact, a primitive diocesan newspaper.

Kate Conway came to know many of the Sisters as she covered stories about the orphanages and schools and, in 1875 she asked if she could live at Nazareth for a time. She continued to edit the *West End Journal* and, in exchange for her room and board, she taught English to the older girls and kept the convent records current.

Kate was very bright, committed to her work in journalism and education, and down-to-earth. She stayed at Nazareth, a welcome and vibrant part of the community there, until 1878, when the Buffalo diocesan paper, *The Catholic Times,* merged with her little *West End Journal.* She went to Buffalo to join their staff.[10]

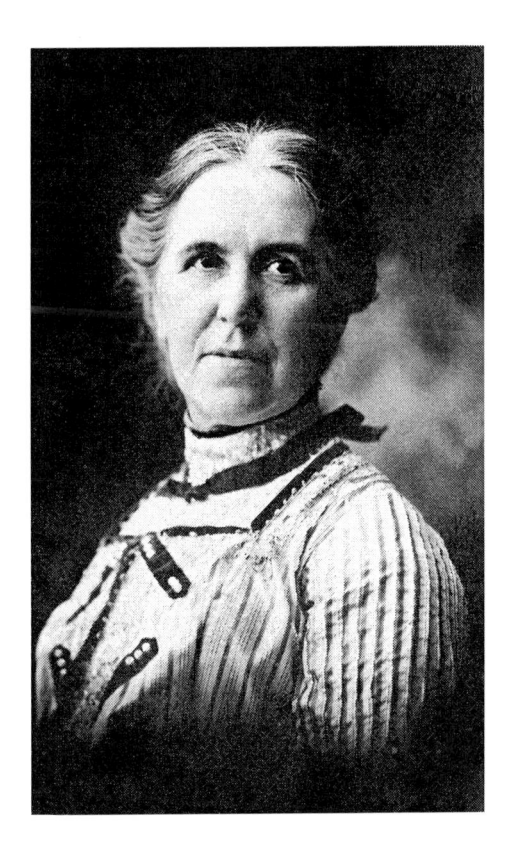

*Katherine Conway, in later years, was well known as a journalist, editor of the Boston **Pilot** and writer of "Catholic fiction"*

Katherine Conway's three years with the Sisters stood in sharp contrast to Alice Seymour's six-month fiasco. Kate and the Sisters had been young together. She understood them, loved them, appreciated their earnest, if simple, zeal and overlooked their sometimes childish failings. Later she wrote of those days:

Indeed all were young then together, though the few who had reached their 21st year were accounted comparatively elder persons. Much wisdom was expected of them, and I fear disedification now and then resulted when they were surprised in the occasional freakishness of lingering youth.[11]

In other words, these were teenagers who were trying to be adults, and not always succeeding. She describes them with affection and admiration:

What fervent, whole-hearted, unquerying children they were--from 5 A.M. to 9:30 P.M.--studying and working, with fully five hours in the chapel..., practicing rigorous self-denial...and withal as merry as children on a holiday![12]

Alice Seymour did not see them that way. Later that year she would write to Bishop McQuaid:

It was a mistaken kindness in Rev. Mother to place a mere *secular* boarder in the midst of the Sisters. I loved them and, older, with more experience, seeing their faults, I longed to raise these young women to my own standards of womanly dignity and calm intellectual tastes.[13]

She suggested that her problem with them stemmed from the fact that she had been instructed in the faith "more intellectually than it is well for a woman to be."[14] It is more likely that many of the less-impressed Sisters had caught on to her odd gentility, affected manners and implied superiority and had seen her influence on the young ones. It was never clear just why she had come.

That she was a talented musician was never a question. Hard-working, well educated, proficient in seven languages, and a teacher for many years, she wanted to influence these young women in ways of the world she knew. She had a grand piano in the back parlor and was already practicing by 5:30 when the Sisters came down for morning prayers. She trained the Sisters' choir and worked with individuals she felt had promise. The novices and young professed Sisters were fascinated, and Sister Berchmans, by then the novice mistress (something of a *grande dame* herself, and still homesick for Belgium) felt a kinship with her European manners.

There was about her the air of a fragile, failed aristocratic lady, once wealthy and now forced to earn a common living. She continued to gather her young admirers about her, calling herself their "1/4 Sister." But her presence, though a source of pride and a drawing card for the Academy, became more and more divisive among the Sisters there. When she left that summer, it was with great bitterness.

But petty squabbles paled when the next blow fell. One steamy evening in late June, teachers, students, parents, friends, the bishop and a score of interested priests gathered for Nazareth Academy's graduation. After the ceremony, mothers and Sisters scurried around the flower-filled reception hall, arranging and serving refreshments; fresh-faced graduates received the proud glances of family and friends; the Sisters, undoubtedly, thought of vacation and Hemlock Lake.

The terrible testing

Bishop McQuaid took Mother Stanislaus aside. He had received word from *L'Ecole St. Andre* that Sister Seraphine O'Kane was dying. "Quick consumption" they had called it. He had purposely waited until after the graduation to tell her, because he wanted to be sure that things were in order before she left for Belgium. She was to leave for Belgium the next day, he told her, to bring Seraphine home. She was to take Sister Berchmans with her, he said, because Berchmans was Belgian; she could handle the practical problems of language, currency, customs and directions. It was settled, he said. He had made all the arrangements.

This was a test for his "obedient child." She was

stunned. Seraphine was dying. He had received this terrible news, not she. He had decided to keep it from her until now. He had decided how and when and with whom she would respond. He had arranged everything.

Deeply grieved, Mother Stanislaus and Sister Berchmans boarded the train for New York City the next evening. There was one arrangement that McQuaid knew nothing about. Mother Stanislaus had wired her friend Baptista Hanson in Brooklyn, to tell her they were coming. She needed a friend and knew that Baptista would respond.

Baptista was waiting for them when their train pulled into the station the next morning. Their ship did not sail until evening, so she took them to St. John's in Brooklyn. They could rest; they could wait out the hours together; they could talk. Baptista saw them safely to the *Nederland,* the steamer that would carry them to Antwerp.

The journey that Sisters Seraphine and deSales had made to Belgium two years before had been dangerous. This one was merely miserable. The *Nederland* was small, though it still retained the typical classes: first, second and steerage. (Sister Berchmans, embarrassed that they had first class accommodations, is quick to say in her account that they had not chosen it, that their passage had been booked by diocesan officials.) The staterooms were tiny; it was already a hot summer; there was only a single small deck for passengers' use.

Both of them became seasick the first day and stayed seasick for the entire voyage. "We remained on deck as long as we could," Sister Berchmans recalls, "for the air was much better than in the sickening, dirty cabins."[15] If first class was as unbearable as she describes it, God help the people in steerage!

They were barely off the ship at Antwerp (resisting the urge, no doubt, to kiss the solid ground), when they heard of President Garfield's assassination. For Mother

Stanislaus, who had never traveled abroad, such news of home seemed surreal as she looked around her. They walked through an open air market and she was enchanted by the colorful, old fashioned costumes of the Flemish peasants who had come to the city to sell their produce. Berchmans could not convince her that all Belgians did not dress like that.

Monsignor DeRegge's sister, a Sister of Charity, was superior of St. Vincent's Convent in Antwerp. She welcomed them warmly. The next day Berchmans met her sister and they went to visit their father in their childhood home, a distance away.

Mother Stanislaus was happy just to stay at St. Vincent's. She had never really regained all her strength since her sickness; she still felt the sting of Father O'Hare's treatment of her; Alice Seymour had had Nazareth in an uproar the past few months; there had been that awful ocean voyage. And dear Seraphine was dying. She was only twenty-one, and she was dying. Things seemed out of her hands, out of her control. She could use some time alone.

This was Sister Berchmans' first time home since she had entered the community. It was bittersweet. She was frustrated. "It was a hurried, fatiguing journey by coach and stage," she wrote, "and having to be back in Antwerp two days later, we had no opportunity of seeing our friends."[16] She well knew that she would not be back for a long time, maybe never. This trip had been totally unexpected. She was only here at all because the bishop had decided that she would be useful. As soon as she returned to Antwerp, she and Mother Stanislaus left for Bruges.

They were not prepared to see Seraphine. Skeleton-thin, bones showing through her skin, her eyes dark and set deep in their sockets, weak and scared, she only wanted to go home. She was barely holding on.

And poor deSales had been courageously tending her for weeks, watching her friend deteriorate by the day. She was weak with relief when she saw them.

They set out for home the next day. The trip back rivaled the first in pure misery. As they left the harbor, they had a near-collision with another ship. During the voyage: one of the crew fell from the main mast and broke his neck; a woman died in steerage; an engineer was killed when he fell to the deck from a high place; and a little child died, suddenly. The food had spoiled in the heat, so they ate only what was in tins. The three took shifts, around the clock, to look after Seraphine who could not leave the stifling cabin. They arrived in Rochester, finally, on August 4. They had been gone six weeks.

At Nazareth the Sisters got word of their arrival in New York and began scurrying around to get together a spontaneous homecoming. They had hoped to have organized a huge welcome, with drama, music, recitations, and original poetry composed for the occasion--the works (the usual) - but there was no time. Alice Seymour had left, hurt and anger in her wake. Things were tense at Nazareth.

Many of the Sisters were still at Hemlock, where they had spent much of July. It had been a full summer. The bishop had done a great deal of entertaining this year. He liked to show off his community to his Episcopal friends. Sometimes they did not perform to standards. July 12 was his anniversary, and he had the Sisters serve his dinner party. After dinner, he called one of the Sisters aside and gave her "a lecture about awkwardness and shyness...for not saluting in the proper way ecclesiastical dignitaries."[17]

He wanted them to be lively, but not forward; bright but not smart; humble, but not shy; self-possessed but subservient. He was not an easy man to please.

A week later, he received a long letter signed "Maria Alexia Veronica Seymour de St. Maur" saying that she had "left Nazareth with contempt in (her) heart." She accused an (unnamed) priest of spreading (unnamed) rumors about her and some of the Sisters of complicity with him in smearing her good name. With high drama she declared that "Six months in that Convent taught me more of the low minded petty jealousies, deceitfulness and untruthfulness of women than all the intrigues and diplomacy at the Austrian court."

McQuaid, straightforward and unsentimental, must have flinched at the hyperbole and shrugged at her Big Finish: "With Protestants and Catholics both against me, I can discover but three means of escape: death, insanity or infidelity. Into which shall I fling myself?"[18]

There is no further mention of Alice Seymour in community records or evidence of further correspondence with the bishop. The unease she left in her wake made the Belgian homecomings even more welcome.

Seraphine was comfortable, happy to be home. Mother Stanislaus knew that everyone wanted to know what had happened. She visited every house. Hemlock was her last stop. Bishop Corrigan was visiting when she came. He sat on the verandah and watched the Sisters run to meet her. He compared her arrival to "a lump of sugar covered with flies."[19] It was a crude analogy. But Corrigan was a close friend of Bishop McQuaid. Perhaps he was privy to the plans McQuaid had for the community by year's end.

The Sisters would have ignored the put-down implicit in Corrigan's inelegant remark. Once they were alone, Mother Stanislaus regaled them with their adventures. It had been the first time she had been away from the community and they had felt her absence.

Once the school term began, things normalized.

They now staffed fourteen (growing) schools and this work took all their energy and attention.

Seraphine held her own, even rallied for a time, but on November 3, 1881 she died. She was twenty-one.

Just before Christmas Mother Stanislaus received a letter from the bishop, telling her to gather all the superiors together for a meeting:

...you will call (them) together during Christmas week, the sooner the better, that I may speak to them. Those Superiors, the present officers of the Community, including the Mistress of Novices and past Mistresses of Novices, will have a voice in deciding on the merits of the candidates for profession. ...Read over your Constitutions and Rules and see that all the officers required by them are called to this work. It is specially enjoined that in every house there shall be a Monitor whose duties are laid down in said rules. A very strict compliance with the rules is essential for the welfare of a large and growing community. Other remarks will be made at another time.
B., Bp. of Rochester[20]

His plans were starting to take shape.

9   FOR REASONS BEST KNOWN TO HIMSELF

January 1, 1882 opened an eventful year in the history of our community. Suffice it to say in advance that in the most trying events of a religious, it were well to remember the words of the inspired prophet: 'He that watcheth over Israel slumbereth not, nor sleeps'.

Annals, Sisters of St. Joseph of Rochester

The profession that the Bishop was so concerned about was that of novices Leander Curry, Hilda Quirk, Claudia O'Rourke and Herman McGuignan. It was Sister Herman who was the real concern, and her "case" became a new battleground.

Sister Herman McGuignan became a postulant with the Sisters of St. Joseph after leaving a Canandian community. No one knew just why she had left the other group, but her time on Jay Street had been stormy, exasperating and a bit bizarre. The Blessed Virgin, she told them, had come to her in a vision telling her to join the Sisters of St. Joseph. She often spoke of visions and revelations that had come to her since she was a child. Bernadette Soubirous, the visionary of Lourdes, was the object of popular devotion at this time. Miss McGuignan was obviously highly suggestible.

She told the Sisters that she was nearly blind, but when she realized that this would be an impediment to her receiving the habit, she was suddenly cured during meditation one winter morning. All was quiet in the chapel, as others prayed (or dozed, which was often the case). All at once Herman jumped from the pew shouting, "My God! I can see!" Our Lady of Lourdes had cured her, she said.

For some reason, her superiors gave her the benefit of the doubt and allowed her to become a novice. During her novitiate her "visions" continued. A statue of Mary, missing from the community room, was found next to her bed. Soon after that it disappeared altogether and a similar statue (taken, they found, from St. Patrick's Orphanage) appeared at the back gate. Pieces of the first one turned up in the furnace. Mary, she said, had told her that she must make profession of vows.

No more benefit of a doubt. Sister Herman had to go.

But she did not go gently. She insisted that the Blessed Virgin wanted her to be professed. Her confessor, believing that she was a true visionary, a chosen soul, insisted as well. Mother Stanislaus, who knew delusions when she saw them, would not budge. Sister Herman would not be admitted to vows. Not now, not ever. Father Saltig took the matter to higher authority.

Sister Berchmans was the Novice Mistress at this time and probably closest to the whole painful affair. She wrote:

> Sister Herman...pretended that the Blessed Virgin would help her and that without fail she was going to make her vows. But Mother Stanislaus firmly opposed it, notwithstanding the protestations and supplications of our confessor, Rev. Father Saltig, CSSR, who was strongly in favor of Sister Herman and believed every word she told him.[1]

Mother Stanislaus called together the group the bishop had requested though, according to the Constitution of that time, there was no need to include all the superiors in the community, as he had directed.[2] He seemed to want as broad a base as possible in deciding on the candidates. He was not going to allow Mother Stanislaus to make this decision on her own. It was a serious thing to disregard the advice of a confessor. McQuaid spoke to the group first; then they were free to judge the fitness of the candidates according to their rule.

On January 6, 1882, Sisters Hilda, Leander, and Claudia professed their vows. Herman stayed on for a few weeks; then Father Saltig steered her into another order in the Midwest. She returned almost at once, saying that she could not find the convent he had sent her to, and that the Blessed Virgin wanted her here. Consistency was one of Sister Herman's virtues. For some reason, the Sisters of St. Patrick's Orphanage took her in, but by February 23 she was officially dismissed.

Sister Berchmans, looking back on those nerve-wracking days, saw this as the beginning of the end of things-as-they-were. Something had happened in the community that could not be changed or taken back:

Whether or not these things were connected with the subsequent disturbances in the community during the spring and summer of that year, it is hard to tell. Excitement had now found it way into our hitherto peaceful community, and it is not improbable that among so large a number of members some were found who delighted in stirring up the fires of excitement and eagerness for change. The result will be told in its own time...[3]

Mother Stanislaus had, it seems, taken too much authority to herself, had influenced others to go against the judgment of a priest. There was a new division in the community.

Though Mother Stanislaus had won this round, McQuaid continued to be the arbiter of community disputes and to make final decisions in serious problems that involved professed Sisters. The community had grown to almost two hundred by 1882. There were bound to be personnel problems: interpersonal, spiritual, psychological, even, in one case, legal. Petitions, apologies, flatteries, explanations, complaints - all landed on his desk and he dealt with his "obedient children" as he saw fit.

After the profession, Mother Stanislaus went to Brooklyn for a few days. She needed to sort things out, and Baptista could always help her see things more clearly. When she got home, she heard that Mother Agnes Spencer was seriously ill in Erie. She went right away.[4]

So much had happened in the twenty-two years since Bishop Timon removed Agnes Spencer from her office, forcing her to find her way elsewhere. Mother Stanislaus remembered that time so well, remembered the pain of losing her, the confusion in the community and the fear of questioning the authority of the bishop in removing this pioneer, their founder, their friend. Mother Stanislaus remembered how the people in Dunkirk had talked about Agnes, had missed her. And then she looked at the Erie community that she had founded when she left. It was

113

growing, even flourishing.

Now Margaret Leary was middle-aged and chafing under the yoke of another bishop. Agnes Spencer had been her first "mother" and in many ways her role model. Agnes' life said to her:

> Nothing is permanent. No place is home forever.
> Go where you are useful. Use your gifts.
> New life can be born out of pain.
> Don't be held down.
> Trust your own instincts.
> Claim your own authority.

Such sentiments were uncommon in nineteenth century women. The suffragettes and some early feminist writers may have made some inroads in encouraging independent thinking, but by and large it would not have occurred to a woman to question her place in the scheme of things or to engage in such self-reflection.

Agnes was still stable when Mother Stanislaus arrived in Erie. Perhaps they had time to say good-bye. The annals record only that in March Mother Stanislaus went to Erie for her funeral.

A quiet jubilee

Valentine's Day 1882 had been Mother Stanislaus' silver jubilee. Ordinarily, a Reverend Mother's jubilee would be a time of huge preparation, of far-flung invitations, of great common rejoicing. Ordinarily, such an event would take place in a bedecked motherhouse chapel or, if that were too small, at the Cathedral. The bishop, flanked by priests from all the parishes where the Sisters served, would celebrate a special Mass; all the stops would be out on the organ; the air would be heavy with the perfume of dozens of flowers. Ordinarily, everyone touched by the life of the jubilarian would be there: civic leaders, representatives from other religious communities, schoolchildren, orphans, parishioners, her family, friends and two hundred Sisters of St. Joseph.

By the time of Mother Stanislaus' jubilee, things had already begun to come undone. She wanted no part of a wide celebration. She wanted only to go quietly back to Canandaigua, where she had begun; she wanted to have an ordinary Mass in the church with whomever was there; she wanted to remember, to recapture, to be immersed in the beginnings.

On February 13 she went to Canandaigua and stayed overnight with the Sisters at St. Mary's. The people in the parish had gotten wind of the occasion, obviously by way of a leak from the convent, and were in church when she arrived for morning Mass. The pastor, Father English (with whom she had had the dispute over salaries in 1870) celebrated the Mass. A young priest friend of hers, Father William Morrin, was at his side.

An article in the *Ontario Messenger* the next week described the low-key celebration:

> The congregation that gathered in St. Mary's Church to do her honor was proof positive of the warm place she occupies in the hearts and affections of the people. Indeed, had it been known to the people of the surrounding country that such a celebration was to take place, the Church would not have contained the numbers that would have been present to give expression to the respect and regard which they have always held and still hold for her. But her humility prevented this, as few, if any, knew of it outside the town itself.[5]

Father Morrin gave the only speech, a short talk at the end of Mass, "giving an outline of this valiant woman's sacrifices and success, congratulating her on both, and praying that she may live to celebrate her golden jubilee, grace and success attending her even to the end."[6]

Rochester was not a peaceful city in 1882. Four hundred of the four hundred fifty workers at Cunningham's carriage factory walked out on strike on January 28. Management all around the city took nervous note. They fought back by forming the Employers' Protection Union to oppose trade unions that were beginning to gain too much strength.

A small pox epidemic prompted the first mass vaccination program for 30,000 frightened Rochesterians.

But a new age began that year, with the coming of the first electric lights.

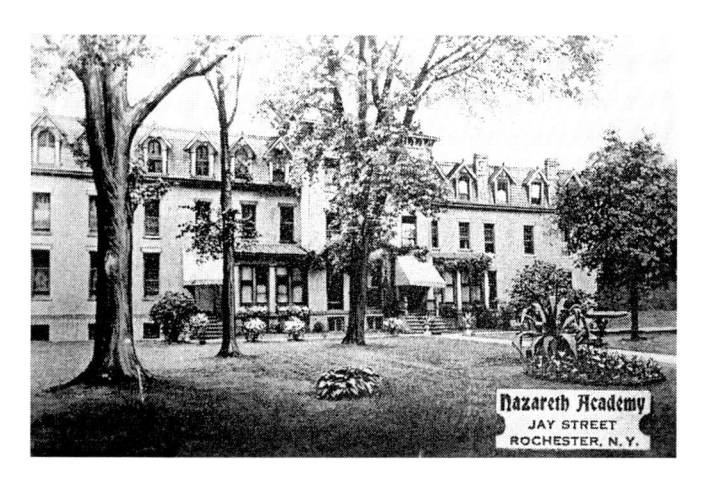

The Jay Street motherhouse

There were still more renovations to be done at the Jay Street property. Once the strikes were over and tradesmen went back to work, Mother Stanislaus began accepting bids. On April 22, she dashed off a note to the bishop:

I here send you the offers of the different builders. They tell me that building materials will be higher next year and, as the strikes of masons

and carpenters are ended and the wages decided upon for this season, I think we had better build if you give us permission...We will not be obliged to borrow but $5000. I will call on you after dinner.
Most respectfully,
M. Stanislaus[7]

"Most respectfully," not "Your obedient child" or "obedient servant" or obedient-anything this time. She planned to build and she would build. The visit, she thought, was merely a formality. The letter gives a plan for the future. She did not know that in a month's time she would have no power to make any decisions for the community's future.

Once things started happening, they happened quickly. After dinner that evening Mother Stanislaus walked over from Nazareth to the bishop's residence. It was late April and, in Rochester, that means that spring, though in the air, teases with balmy-then-chilly breezes, lingering sun, unexpected cold, broken promises. It has been known to snow in April.

Her reception that evening was anything but warm. There would be no more construction at Nazareth. Later that year, McQuaid would make it clear that it had never been *his* intention that Jay Street remain the motherhouse, and he wanted no more expense incurred in changing or expanding it.[8]

Perhaps it was at this meeting that Mother Stanislaus informed him that many of the Sisters did not wish to spend their vacation time at the Hemlock cottage.[9] There were those who still loved going there, but a significant number found oppressive his constant presence and scrutiny, his using them in serving and entertaining his guests, his insistence on using even their leisure time for even more study. She may have even had another place in mind for a summer home.[10]

Perhaps it was at this meeting that he told her of his plans to replace her. At any rate, she knew it well enough by mid-May. On May 15, Bishop McQuaid sent a letter to all of the houses of the Sisters of St. Joseph:

It is now nearly fourteen years since this Community of the Sisters of St. Joseph began its work as an independent organization in the diocese of Rochester. During these years the Community has become a large and flourishing one...

So far the direction of the Community has been in the hands of Mother Stanislaus who had ably and successfully managed the important and responsible task confided to her judgment and zeal. But the time has come when it seems expedient to bring the government of the community more in harmony with the spirit of the rules under which it exists. The rules prescribe that Superiors shall hold office for three years, although the same Superior may be elected and re-appointed.

He went on, quoting their *Constitution* on the procedure for the election of a General Superior: The election will be on Tuesday after Ascension Day. Each Sister shall pray for guidance (even the prayers for guidance are prescribed: offering of Communion on the Sunday within the octave and a daily *Veni Creator* - a magic formula.). No conversations about the election can take place among them. On the appointed day, each Sister, after Holy Communion, writes the names of three Sisters "best suited in her judgment and according to her conscience most capable of filling the office of General Superior for the next term." She places her votes in an envelope and gives it to her local superior who, in turn, gives it to the bishop. The vote is given "to secure for the community the superior best fitted to carry on its good work, to be a source of edification to her fellow Sisters, and to further the ends for which the Community has been instituted." He ended:

You will readily appreciate the importance of your wise selection in effecting a change in the government of your Community. Much depends upon the freedom of the Sisters in giving an unbiased expression of judgment with regard to the Sisters best adapted by their virtues, prudence, experience and ability to rule over a Congregation large and growing as is that of the Sisters of St. Joseph of Rochester. I trust that the plan here proposed will secure this freedom.[11]

He never asked them for an opinion about whether a change was needed; he only asked them for some names. And, in the end, it was a moot point.

The end of a friendship, the end of an era

What had happened? Sister Stanislaus had been his own choice for superior in 1868, when he put into motion his plan for a diocesan Sisterhood. He had seen something in her - a kindness, a simplicity, a natural leadership, a certain malleability - that made him believe that she would serve the role (and him) competently.

But he could not have predicted the astounding growth of the community in fourteen years; nor did he take into account the fact that people change. The woman who was Mother Stanislaus in 1882 was far different from the eager, immature, well-intentional twenty-seven-year-old of his original choice.

For years she had fought for just wages, or any wages at all, for the Sisters' work in the schools. He simply told them to keep on sacrificing, to be more frugal and to pull together.

He wanted the Sisters to have a first-rate education, but it was they who had to earn the money to pay for it.

He objected to all the improvements and expansions she was making at Nazareth. She was forced to become "creative" with money. (More than once, amounts were transferred, as "a loan", from the St. Mary's Asylum account to Nazareth Convent.) She was coming to resent his power over all aspects of their lives. She was starting to claim her own authority in the community, independent of his. This change had come gradually, but by 1882 her independence had become a stumbling block to his plans.

Even before he sent the letter, the community had already been in something of turmoil. Sister Berchmans had resigned as Mistress of Novices and the bishop blamed Mother Stanislaus, accusing her of prejudice against Berchmans. This makes little sense. Berchmans was a strong support to Mother Stanislaus; there was between them a genuine respect and affection that is evident in Berchmans' own words in the Annals; they had a special bond since their shared ordeal when they went to Belgium to get Seraphine.

But Mother Stanislaus could do little to please McQuaid at that time. The cards were stacked against her. Berchmans' wrote at once to the bishop, to clear things up:

> It was at my own request that Rev. Mother allowed me to resign the office of Mistress of Novices. Not finding myself capable of discharging it properly, I asked her to give it to one more able and more worthy. That Rev. Mother was ever prejudiced against me, is, I believe, a misunderstanding. She was always kind to me, and I feel most grateful towards her, as I do towards all my benefactors.[12]

That same day Mother Stanislaus wrote him a letter which, unfortunately, does not survive. It must have been an angry one, because this is what he shot back at her:

> Rev. Mother,
> I am sorry you wrote the letter you sent me yesterday. When you become cooler you also will regret that you wrote it.
> What I propose to do for the welfare of your community shall be done according to my best judgment and conscience. It is your duty and that of your Sisters to pray that God may guide me in my decision.
> Of two things I feel sure: 1. I have the best interest of the Community at heart; 2. I permit no prejudice or personal feeling to influence me. You can rest assured that I have no thought of permitting anything to be

done under any circumstance...that will be unworthy of the respect and honor due to you and your long service.

I had looked to you for assistance in carrying on the government of the Community, but you write in your letter as though all such assistance would be withheld...You will please to hold office until I change you...Begging God to be with you. Yours sincerely in Christ,

+Bernard, Bp. of Rochester[13]

The "Begging God to be with you" is almost-tender, almost-vulnerable, almost-regretful. Their correspondence from this day on is laced with restrained pain like this - the pain of friends who are no longer friends, trying to speak to each other, unable to bridge the new space between them, unable to penetrate the stony silence that marks their relationship.

They continued to wound each other: he with authoritarian high-handedness, innuendo, scolding, cold disregard for her feelings; she with stubbornness, refusal to disappear quietly, thinly disguised defiance, verbal barbs and - she knew this drove him wild - constant changing of her mind and plans. The rift was irreparable.

The community was deeply divided (though tradition holds that most of the Sisters were strongly pro-Mother Stanislaus and near revolt at the Bishop's ultimatum). They disregarded the mandate about not discussing the election. In fact, many (if not most) were determined to send in blank ballots or ballots with only Mother Stanislaus' name. She heard of it and wrote:

As our good Bishop has thought fit to make a change in the government of the Community, it is your duty as good and obedient religious to submit in all humility and to show no opposition of any kind, as all authority comes from God.

My wish is that in returning the tickets you should act according to conscience. Do not be influenced by the natural affection you bear to anyone. Do no return the blanks unfilled, as this would give offense to the Bishop. Surely out of such a large Community, three persons can be found to fill my office. If, in your judgment, there are not three persons, then write the names of two or one.

This change will not deprive me of watching over the Community and its interests, which are the dearest objects in my life. I would be a miserable religious indeed if I could not bear it with resignation and conformity to God's will. I will try to make myself happy in whatever work may be assigned to me. I have always tried to do my duty as well as I know how. None of us can do all things perfectly.

Now, my dear Sisters, pray that God may direct your choice. I trust that as good religious you will try to be satisfied with the one the Bishop appoints. Show the obedience and respect due to her office and love and obey your rules.

My beloved Sisters, I ask your prayers that God may give me humility and meekness.

Yours affectionately in Christ,
M. Stanislaus[14]

The "election" took place on schedule. The Sisters sealed their ballots and sent them to the bishop. On May 29 he announced that Sister Agnes Hines would be their new superior. Everyone knew that this was an appointment, not an election. The bishop had every right to appoint whomever he wished. The Sisters knew that their votes would probably have no bearing on the outcome, but they were satisfied to have made their statement.

Sister Agnes was a reluctant appointee and begged to be spared the burden of office. She was only too well aware of the special problems that she would face trying to unify a very scattered community.

There are any number of interpretations of this event. The question that remains about it is not *what* happened but *why*. The bishop's explanation that Mother Stanislaus' replacement was mandated by the rule was true but obviously a red herring. Mother Agnes Hines, whose appointment was supposed to have begun a regularization of terms of office, remained in the office for thirty-nine years! It was not the rule McQuaid was concerned about, but the future usefulness and survival of the community in the diocese.

He simply used the time-honored excuse: "It's the law."

Women are familiar with that particular phrase: "You can't vote. It's the law." "You can't own property. It's the law." And, in the Church, "You can't be ordained. It's the law." And when they ask: "Who makes these laws? Who decides?", they are met with stony silence and polemics. They are scolded or shamed or lightly mocked. They are "too emotional" or they are "irrational" or they "don't understand."

Bishop McQuaid spoke at the Cathedral one evening, two years later. "Woman owes the position she occupies today," he said, "to the Catholic Church. It was the Catholic Church that raised her from the degradation to which she had been consigned and placed her in the exalted position she now occupies."[15]

He believed this. He also believed that women were capable of real, if limited, contributions. He cheered the suffragettes on. *Of course* women should vote. He held that women made the finest teachers and healers. He appreciated their intellectual gifts and wanted "his" Sisters to be well educated, their talents fully realized.

But he would not, could not relinquish his grip on their destiny. The task before them was serious and clear: the Catholic schools. There was no room, no time for maverick behavior, for playing games with his authority. Their task, he was to tell them, was to help the clergy. In a conference he told them:

Now you Sisters can never dream of aspiring to anything like the position of the priest. Whoever made that choice it was not man; it was God...Your merit depends in great abundance in cooperating with the priests in the work they have in saving souls...especially...the instruction of the young.[16]

He would often compare their lives with

martyrdom. He encouraged them to give everything for the cause of Catholic education:

> In the future, as in the past, go on with generous spirits, go down to your graves like the martyrs, not running away from the danger but right on the field of battle...Go on with the good work, helpers of the clergy...[17]

All of the written accounts of this time gloss over the possible *whys*. Katherine Conway, who as a lifelong friend of both McQuaid and Agnes Hines must have known something of the circumstances, concentrated on the effect Mother Stanislaus' removal had on the Sisters:

> The changing of a beloved Mother Superior is always a sore trial in the life of a young community, and when, as in this case, she was the first, a woman of rare charm and magnetism, having been to some...the only mother they ever knew, the gravity of the crisis can be realized.[18]

McQuaid visited the grieving community and, came close to admitting he may have handled it badly: "My shoulders are broad," he said. "If there is blame, and I blame myself, I will bear it."[19]

Sister Berchmans got out of it with her usual circumspection. In the *Annals* she stated simply that "for reasons best known to himself, our Rt. Rev. Bishop and Superior resolved to make a change in the governance of the community," adding only that he "met with a great deal of opposition."[20]

All of the records are silent about this critical time. There is no revealing correspondence, either in McQuaid's voluminous papers or in the community archives. McQuaid, who saved scraps of papers, handwritten drafts of speeches, bills from builders, orders for vegetables from Excelsior Farms, anniversary greetings, and letters from hundreds of people, saved not a word about this incident which obviously concerned him deeply.

The Congregation's *Annals*, so detailed and exact in other matters, are mute. A total of fifteen pages are missing from the bound annals - sliced clean with a razor or knife. These pages come just before or after stories of: Father James Early's departure from the diocese, Sister Herman's dismissal and Mother Stanislaus' removal from office. Someone, obviously, had been cast in an unfavorable light and a self-appointed censor took it upon herself to bowdlerize the official story.

Community lore is full of old stories and rumors, whispers of Mother Stanislaus' unseemly behavior (being seen in an open carriage, or driving the buggy for the Sisters instead of hiring a man to do it), of her continued correspondence with James Early, of her accepting a vacation house from a benefactor. None seems serious enough to warrant the treatment she got from Bernard McQuaid.

The best clues come in the correspondence and the council meeting minutes of the months that followed.

10 IF YOU WOULD JUST LEAVE ME ALONE

I promise your Lordship that I will never again mention your name whether for good or evil if you will just leave me alone.

Mother Stanislaus to Bishop McQuaid

McQuaid wasted no time in establishing his policy. On June 2, only four days after the appointment of Mother Agnes, he called a council meeting with the new officers. He made clear to them that he would preside over council meetings as often as he could and that his voice would always be the deciding factor in their deliberations. According to the minutes of that meeting: "After exhorting the Sisters to fulfill zealously and in the spirit of obedience the duties of their respective charges, the Rt. Rev. Bishop decides."[1]

Having made that clear, he was ready to begin again. The council met again on June 5, this time without the Bishop, with a four-item agenda. Two questions, permission for a Sister to attend a relative's funeral and the dismissal of a novice, were routine and easily dispensed with. The other items were hot potatoes.

First, what to do with Mother Stanislaus? She had asked to begin a new mission in Boston. Should they let her go? Father Michael O'Brien from Lowell, Massachusetts, had written to McQuaid as early as 1875, asking for some Sisters of St. Joseph to run a House of Protection for unemployed, homeless women.[2] Mother Stanislaus had visited there and at a similar place in Boston and had expressed an interest in this work. O'Brien had been impressed with her and with the work her community was doing in Rochester.

At the time McQuaid would not hear of his Sisters leaving the diocese or engaging in any new work. He needed them all. But Mother Stanislaus did not forget the offer and, when she knew she would be leaving her office, she contacted Father O'Brien and tentatively accepted.

The council decided that "under the present circumstances it would be best not to oppose the opening of the...mission."[3] They did not know just what to do with her, and this was a good solution. It seemed best to give her whatever she wanted. The tone of the decision, however, was tight and irritable. Mother Stanislaus was not fading away quietly. Her presence since the election made them uncomfortable; it would be a relief if she simply left the diocese.

The other problem they addressed holds a clue to some of the McQuaid's anger toward Mother Stanislaus:

The Rt. Rev. Bishop having heard that some community members are opposed to the Sisters' spending their vacation at Hemlock, wishes to have this matter settled by the council, his aim being the good of the community, not the disturbance of religious discipline.[4]

Dissatisfaction with the arrangement at Hemlock

was a slap in the bishop's face, a rejecting of his hospitality. But more than that, his bringing it before the council gives credence to the story that Mother Stanislaus indeed did have access to another summer residence. According to that story, a benefactor had given her a large country villa for a vacation house for the Sisters. McQuaid had insisted that she give the deed to him and she refused. The final straw.

The story is plausible. The council minutes make it clear that some Sisters were unhappy with the Hemlock set-up, whether because of distance or danger in getting there, or the constant intrusion of Bishop McQuaid into their every move. If someone had offered a possible alternative, Mother Stanislaus would certainly have accepted it.

At this time, McQuaid needed money. He had already begun collecting for his seminary, and was not encouraged by the amounts he had received so far. He could have realized a good deal of seed money from the sale of good property. In April and May of 1882, he tried to sell a large piece of property and had trouble doing it because he did not have "clear title."[5] The matter was settled in June 1882. By then he had made it clear that the Sisters would not be going anywhere but Hemlock for vacation.

Not surprisingly, the new council agreed with him "that Hemlock cottage situated as it is in a healthy, quiet region, presents many advantages for spending vacation, and no more dangers than any other place."[6] They stayed with Hemlock. There would be no more deviations.

McQuaid called yet another meeting on June 7. He was furious. He had called them together:

...to settle some difficulties occasioned by the disagreement of parties in the election of the new general superior; that false rumors...have given much disedification and that, since moderation and kindness have failed, the refractory members shall be forbidden to keep up correspondence with the former superior.[7]

Further, Mother Stanislaus had first accepted the mission in Boston and a day later changed her mind. She was toying with him and he knew it. He told the council that he withdrew his permission for opening the mission and that he himself would deal with Mother Stanislaus. He told her to remain at St. Mary's Asylum until he gave her an assignment. Her rebellious supporters were not to communicate with her there.

He ended his tirade with a familiar theme: unnecessary travel and visiting are a waste of time and money; they were to stay home and economize. They could then begin saving for his dream for them: a motherhouse in the country.[8]

He was giving some permission for travel, however. Sister Adelaide Carberry, a well-respected older member of the community, had become ill from the stress of the difficult weeks before the election. She went to Brooklyn to spend some time away from the epicenter. Mother Baptista would understand; she could talk it out with her.

When she arrived home Sister Adelaide wrote the Bishop that she had been sick:

...consequent on the trying ordeal I was put through by the new Superior...Now at my return with a good will to renew my labors in obedience to whoever is placed over me, I am informed that I cannot remain...In God's name, dear Bishop, let me know what I am to do.[9]

McQuaid must have taken her part, because Adelaide Carberry remained in the community until her death in 1922.

The Press: the "deposing" goes public

Enter the media. What had begun as an internal Church matter had become public. On June 8 the Buffalo diocesan paper, *The Catholic Union and Times* reprinted this article from the Rochester *Post Express:*

> A reporter called at the Nazareth Convent on the corner of Jay and Frank Streets in quest of news regarding rumored changes in the management of this important religious and educational institution. The Mother Superior had a natural delicacy in being interviewed personally concerning the matter, and deputized a Sister who was authorized to speak with the scribe. From the latter it was learned that Mother Stanislaus, who for eighteen years past has had charge of the institution, is no longer the Mother Superior. At the recent election held, although all the members of the community of Nazareth voted for her reelection, Bishop McQuaid preferred that a change should be made and installed Sr. Agnes in her place. Mother Stanislaus...established the orphan boys' asylum in this city, and in the same year she became Mother Superior of Nazareth Convent. Since then she has established schools from this convent in almost every village in the diocese, displaying much energy in the important work of educating the young. Eighteen years ago the community of the Sisters of St. Joseph in this city numbered but three members; now it numbers 180.
>
> 'We were all against her removal,' said the Sister who furnished the information, 'and quite a stir was caused in our little community by the Bishop's action. Mother Stanislaus has always been amiable and kind and her disposition and manner of managing affairs here endeared her to everyone.'
>
> It was learned that the deposed Mother Superior has left for St. Joseph's Convent in St. Louis, Mo., accompanied by Sr. Cecelia, a music teacher from the convent who withdrew from it to show her sympathy for Mother Stanislaus. Sr. Agnes, the new Mother Superior, has always resided in Rochester and has been connected with Nazareth Convent for twelve years past.[10]

In "deputizing" a Sister to speak for her to the press, Mother Stanislaus was fighting back in the only way left to her. Typical of newspaper reporting, this story had a mix of true and false information: Mother Stanislaus had indeed been in Rochester since 1864, but not Reverend Mother until the diocese was established in 1868; Sister Cecilia Meehan had obtained permission from Bishop McQuaid to accompany Mother Stanislaus on a visit to Carondelet in the summer, to visit her aunts who were members of the community in St. Louis.[11] The story of her dramatic sympathy gesture made good copy, but the truth is she never left the Rochester congregation.

Then, as now, it seemed best to read newspapers with a healthy skepticism. The unnamed "deputy's" contention that all the members of the community had voted for Mother Stanislaus, or that she had endeared herself to everyone may have been harmless hyperbole, or it may have been calculated to embarrass the bishop.

If it were the latter, it worked beautifully. On June 15, Bishop McQuaid dashed off an angry letter to Bishop Ryan of Buffalo, who had evidently offered McQuaid equal time in the *Catholic Union and Times*.

"I acquit you," McQuaid told the Buffalo bishop, "of any intention to bring contempt on the Bishop of Rochester, but I do not exonerate the editor or manager of the paper."

Rochesterians, he said, ignored the "silly gossip" of the *Post-Express*, and it hurt him that it would be reprinted in a Catholic paper.

"The real harm of this publication," he contended, "is that I am placed by my own diocesan poor people in country places in the light of a despot who is treating humble Sisters with gross injustice. Should I ever care to place myself right before my diocese it will not be through the columns of the 'Catholic Union'"[12]

The fact that Katherine Conway had been the staff member responsible for accepting and printing the article only deepened the wound for McQuaid. They were friends, or so he had thought. The incident caused a rift of silence between them that lasted for four years. He would hear no apology on the matter, no explanation.

It was she, finally, who broke through the silence and wrote to him in 1886. By then she was on the staff of the Boston *Pilot*, well respected in her field, and distanced from the painful events of 1882:

...When the change of Mother Superiors was made at Nazareth, I was aware of the bare fact; but utterly ignorant of preceding or attendant circumstances—had no idea of insubordination, unpleasant publicity or scandal of any sort. I was alone in charge of the paper, the day the *Post Express* paragraph came. It came from Rochester enclosed in a brief note, requesting publication in the next issue. To you, at the scene of the trouble, it may seem hardly possible that to no one at a distance and ignorant of the actual state of affairs, the clipping had no vicious meaning...

The day following publication, I learned the truth. I saw the venom of the paragraph, and the motive that had sought and compassed its production in a Catholic paper. As days went by I saw the position it put you in. I cannot express to you what I felt about it. I offered every reparation in my power. There seemed to be none possible except to hear the blame of having done an ungrateful, treacherous, and sinful thing. Even those who, then I had reason to think were parties to the sending of the paragraph, were loudest in assigning all blame to me...

The whole matter must be a life's regret to me in any case; but if you knew all, I think you would not withhold your pardon nor refuse to see me if the opportunity I hope for comes.[13]

McQuaid finally forgave her what he then believed was her unwitting part in slandering his reputation. But in 1882 he had been far from this forgiving disposition. He concentrated on keeping the cap on any further public displays.

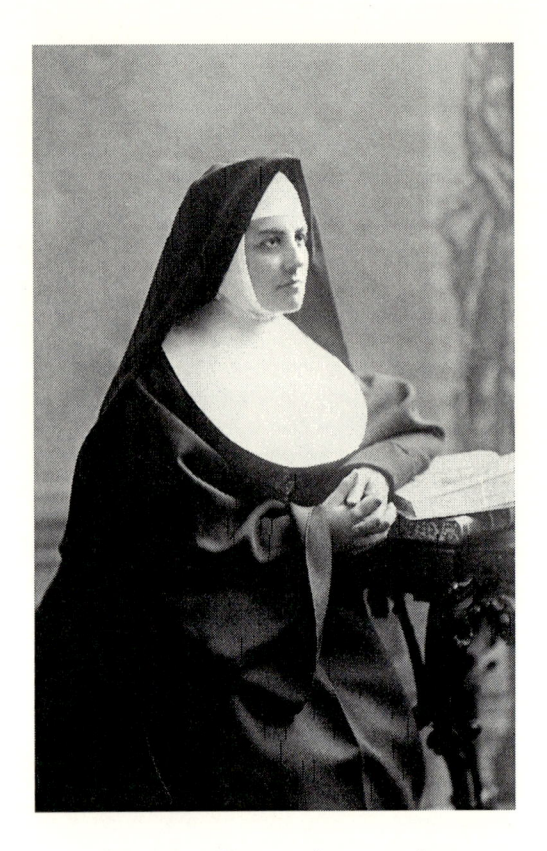

Mother Agnes Hines took over as the new Superior of a troubled and divided community.

All of this was making the new Mother Agnes very uncomfortable. On June 14, 1882 she wrote a frantic note to the bishop:

I am indeed sorry to be obliged to trouble you so soon again. I feel that in the present state of our community I cannot do my duty. Last evening Mother Stanislaus arrived here (Nazareth) and this morning she informed me that her intentions are to remain here...the younger Sisters and novices are completely upset, as Mother has a great deal of influence over them.

You do not have the faintest idea of the state our community is in. I beg of you...to come home this evening if possible and see Mother, also the officers, for I think the sooner things are settled the better for our Community.[14]

He must have managed to get Mother Stanislaus out of town for a while. Perhaps she took that trip to Carondelet. In any case, she was not in Rochester when James Early wrote a cryptic note from Hornellsville on July 5, 1882:

Dear Sister,
I received yours yesterday. I concur in your reasons for not calling at Hornellsville. When you will have arrived in Rochester I will see you at Mrs. Mathews[15] where I will place at your disposal the papers.
I have contracted a sore eye that unfits me to do anything. I can with difficulty read my office and am unable to examine my papers to reach the documents I intended to send you. In the meantime, don't be disheartened. You are right. Go ahead.
Your friend,
JM Early[16]

What these papers were we shall probably never know, but she evidently told him of some plan she was hatching for her future. Certainly she had kept James Early apprised of what was going on. In her problems with the bishop she could have found a sure ally in him.

In August she took a trip to Brooklyn. She had been living at St. Mary's, cut off from friends, knowing that her presence was a problem to some in the community. Her health was breaking down. Despite the bishop's expressed displeasure, she went to visit her friend Baptista. When she returned home, she found out just how displeased he was. She wrote to him:

St. Mary's Orphan Asylum
Sept. 6, 1882
Right Reverend Bishop,

Sister Xavier told me that you sent word to her that I was not to receive Holy Communion till I made repration [sic] for going to Brooklyn. I told you in my letter that I did not understand that you had withdrawn such permission but I will preform[sic] any repration you desired.

Will you please let me know when I am to receive Communion? It is the first time in my life I have been deprived of H. Communion and I can assure you that I have never had a greater trial...I go with some of the other Sisters to Sts. Peter and Paul's to Mass, as the Hospital is so very close, I cannot stay there during the Mass on account of my present state of health...Will you please Right Rev. Bishop to answer this letter or if you grant me an interview I will go to see you.
Your Lordship's most humble servant,
Sr. M. Stanislaus [17]

    In this letter her handwriting is erratic, as are her spelling and grammar. Her ideas are fuzzy. She really was sick and sick at heart. To be deprived of Holy Communion was cruel punishment for her.

    The next day a frustrated council met to discuss a request. "For reasons of health," the minutes say, "Mother Stanislaus has requested of Rev. Mother and the council to obtain for her the Bishop's permission for spending the winter in Florida." [18]

    She had been much in evidence since her return home. As long as she was in Rochester, they knew there would be no peace. Sister Evangelist, the Assistant Superior, thought a change would be a good idea. The minutes state:

The Sisters agree to Sr. Evangelist's opinion that since for the present we do not know any means for changing Mother Stanislaus' feelings, it may be hoped that this stay with other religious of our congregation, who are not concerned with the present disturbance...will work some favorable change.[19]

They asked the bishop to let her go. He was not enthusiastic about the request. He had responded to her letter with some accusations about her Brooklyn visit. Her reply is a mix of assertiveness and feminine manipulation:

September 12, 1882
Right Rev. Bishop,

While in Brooklyn I never met a priest but my confessor. I never spoke of our trouble here to anyone but to my friend, Mother Baptista, and if you should care to hear what I said I shall be very glad to oblige you. I will now return the compliment you gave me in my last letter from you. You hear too many lying stories and unfortunately receive the first one brought without any investigation. I hear many unkind and untruthful things you say of me also. I do not think it very honorable in such a great man as you are to carry on such warfare with a poor, weak little creature like me.
I promise your Lordship I will never again mention your name whether for good or evil if you will just leave me alone.
Asking your Lordship's pardon for anything I either done [sic] or said that may have offended you.
I remain with much respect.
Your obedient servant in Christ,
Sister M. Stanislaus[20]

McQuaid wanted it to be perfectly clear that he did not really approve of her going to Florida, that it was the lesser of two evils. She was doing harm, he claimed, to the Rochester community. He wrote:

At the request of others but against my own judgment and at the risk of being again taunted by you with another "change of mind," I accede to your petition and permit you to spend a year in one of the houses of the Sisters of St. Joseph in the states of Georgia or Florida.

Not wanting her to have any illusions that she had won, he continued:

> I do not grant this permission, be it understood, for the reasons put forth by you...it is not customary for religious to move from one part of the country to another for health's sake. Many never leave the house they once enter until death comes. Nor do I consider that your health needs such a change.

He evidently thought that Episcopal consecration gave him the right to comment on medical questions as well as spiritual.

> I grant the permission...because it is evident that a return to the true spirit of a good religious is not possible where you are, and because your influence over the other Sisters is injurious to them and hurtful to the community as a body. Some unfortunate hallucination has come over your mind that hinders you from seeing the errors of the past.
> When you left for Brooklyn you held in your hand my letter which directed you under obedience to go to St. Mary's Orphan Asylum. You did as you pleased..

In other words, she had defied his house arrest.

> Had you been a good religious you would have...sought advice in the right quarter. In going to Brooklyn you placed yourself under the direction of Sister Baptista whose influence over you has been most unfortunate. She never had a good word to say for any superior. She judges for herself where respect for superiors begins and ends; her measure of obedience is ruled by her own wishes and notions; some of these false principles she has gradually instilled into your mind...

At last he comes out with his real reason. She had removed her neck from the yoke. She had made decisions contrary to his. She was not "obedient."

> You may, when humility finds a place in your heart, return to yourself and become an edifying religious. At present I see no hope of this wished-for change. Perhaps in another part of the country, removed from some who do you no good, God's grace may come back to your soul...When you [indecipherable word] I remove all restrictions with regard to Holy Communion, throwing the responsibility on your own

conscience. While you were keeping up an ill spirit among the Sisters and impeding the work of the community your going to Communion was a scandal. I forbid you to visit Sister Baptista, or to correspond with her.

Begging God to open your eyes to your true state to remove the miserable delusions under which you labor and bestow the graces your soul's salvation needs,

I remain, Very Sincerely in Christ,

+Bernard, Bishop of Rochester[21]

Not wanting to fan the flames any higher, the council decided to appoint Sister Ursula Murphy as Mother Stanislaus' companion to Florida, and to hold a quiet formal reception at Nazareth, so the Sisters could say good-bye. By the end of October the two were in Jacksonville.[22]

Several mission houses were disrupted by one or two "loyalists" bent on making their anger felt, but it is important to know that the administrative controversy did not have total control of the lives and hearts of the individual Sisters.[23] For the most part, they went about their daily work, teaching and caring for the orphans as they had before. The tension was felt mostly at Nazareth and mostly by the members of the new administration who were very much caught in the middle.

The council minutes reveal a group torn, worried, burdened with the responsibility of bringing a divided community together with the least possible disruption of their lives and work. For the community to survive this crisis, they would have to be firm; they would have to continue the ordinary tasks and make the everyday decisions; they would have to put personal feelings aside; they would have to take their lead from the bishop.

Some council members had been close to Mother Stanislaus. Sister Rose Hendrick had worked with her for years at St. Mary's Asylum; Sister Berchmans was a loyal friend; Mother Agnes had been her close associate and assistant.

The Florida "underground"

Mother Stanislaus' attitude didn't help. She had not melted silently away; she had not stepped wordlessly down, head bowed, eyes averted. She had been made to pay for what the bishop considered her lack of "religious spirit." Deprived of her position, cut off from friends, she had begun an underground that continued even while she was in Florida.

In her isolation she resorted to the bizarre. In December, a woman in Auburn received a letter by mistake. On New Year's Eve the council heard about it:

> At Rev. Mother's request Sr. Evangelist gave a reading of a letter, signed Mary Casey and addressed to another Mary Casey. It was received, by mistake...and brought to Sr. Catherine who sent it to Rev. Mother. It is proved to be from Mother Stanislaus and addressed under this borrowed name to Sr. Julia[24], who by it is invited to join Mother Stanislaus in Florida. (She) is told that if her disposition are still the same she should ask the Bishop's obedience for this voyage, and not let herself be talked out of it...Mother Stanislaus adds that she had just sent for her own Sister, Sr. Francis Joseph, that all necessary arrangements for both Sisters have already been made in New York...The reading of this letter makes a painful impression on all the Sisters present, as it shows that Mother Stanislaus' feelings are not changed in the least, and that she still holds secret correspondence with many of our Sisters.[25]

The awkward cloak-and-dagger technique which Mother Stanislaus adopted would be funny if its motivation were not so sad. (She evidently even had Baptista working as an operative in New York!) Her loneliness must have been unbearable. It is telling, too, how these minutes are careful to distance her from them, saying that she "holds secret correspondence with *our* Sisters," as if she were no longer part of them. Neither Sister Julia nor Francis Joseph went to Florida.

Mother Stanislaus must have known that she had burned her bridges in Rochester. With things as they were at home, her presence was only a stumbling block. These painful months had left her empty, exhausted, physically weak and emotionally drained. The Florida Sisters had welcomed her warmly; Mother Sidonie had long been a friend, and was happy to be able to give her some space and time to heal. But she knew it was just a stopover.

In Rochester everything returned to normal. Snow. Study. School. Sacrifice. The bishop wanted two more schools opened by September, in Dansville and Penn Yan. He would have no more talk of expanding their work beyond the diocese or of considering ministries other than the schools. The new superior was in complete accord with this. Candidates for the community would be judged in large measure on their ability to study and teach. Three postulants would enter on St. Joseph's Day and would be ready to go into classrooms by fall. Things seemed peaceful and ordered.

Mother Baptista Hanson died on February 22. Not one word survives about Mother Stanislaus' response to the death of her old friend. Did she travel the long way north from Florida to attend the funeral? How did she bear this fresh loss? It cannot have helped her already fragile state.

We only know that she wrote to McQuaid at that time, asking him if she and Sister Ursula might come home in the spring, six months earlier than he had planned. He became edgy. Her return would be sure to churn things up again. He grumbled a reply:

> In answer to your letter asking permission to leave Florida, etc., I wish to say that this is the worst possible season for a return to the North; that people are now going to Florida to escape the climate of Western New York in the months of March and April...You will therefore stay where you are until the first week of May. When you return there will

be an end to your traveling about, and you will be assigned to some occupation in a fixed place. We shall expect you to give some edification to the community by your spirit of obedience and humility. Many things are known to me now of which I was ignorant when you left for Florida.[26]

She did not, of course, stay where she was. His "no more traveling about" mandate proved ironic; by the time she was through, she would have made traveling a career!

While she was in Florida she had been in contact with two prelates in the mission territories of the West.[27] Bishop Salpointe, the Apostolic Vicar of the Arizona territory, begged her to come to that region and start a mission. Bishop Louis Fink of Leavenworth, Kansas had the same message. They told her about the wonderful climate, the friendly people, the real needs.

They wanted her. She didn't know much about the West. But they wanted her. Her roots were deep in New York State. But they wanted her. She was no longer young. But they wanted her. She had never been strong; the year had taken its toll. But they wanted her. A return to Rochester would mean new fights, more negotiation, constant controversy, sure humiliation. And they wanted her.

She made preparations to go home to Rochester and make plans for the adventure of her life.

11 THEY ARE NOT HERE

When in after years some went back to revisit the old place, it did not seem the same, though it recalled to their minds other merry scenes of years gone by. The lighthearted, cheerful Sisters who caused the mirth were no longer there, and the trees, the hilltops and the lovely lake seemed sorrowfully to ask: 'Whom do you seek? They are not here'.

Annals, Sisters of St. Joseph of Rochester

All the while Mother Stanislaus had been in Florida, some Sisters, most of them from St. Patrick's Asylum, had kept the waters rippling.

Sisters Simplicia Hanlon and Domitilla Gannon asked to join the St. Louis community, because it was "more regular and more united" than Rochester's.[1] Sisters Charles Smith and Antoinette Cuff had both strongly objected to the change of superiors, and they had not kept silent about it. It was almost a relief when they, too, asked for an obedience for St. Louis. The council coolly resolved "not to take further notice of them, and let them leave when they please."[2]

Sister Joseph Teresa McGlynn left Geneva and asked to return to her family. Sister Antonius Vogt, a novice at St. Patrick's, became uneasy as she thought about making her vows that summer. Sister Armella McGrath knew she would have to make a decision soon. Life at St. Patrick's had become stultifying for her.

About fourteen Sisters would leave in the next few months. A few changed their destinations when they found out where Mother Stanislaus was. Their problem was not with religious life in general, but with this new administration in particular.

Mother Stanislaus came home in March, in spite of the bishop's clear command to stay until May. But he probably did not make too much of it, once she told him of her plans. She had accepted Bishop Salpointe's offer. She would go to Arizona and start a new foundation there. She knew there were some Sisters who wanted to go with her-- her two sisters, of course, and others with whom she had been in contact.

McQuaid was only too glad to let her go. It solved some major problems he had anticipated on her return. He would not need to punish, isolate, counsel, scold; he would not need to find some work for her that would both be of use and keep her from influencing the impressionable; he would be able to turn his energy and attention away from her at last and go forward with his plans for the community.

Yes, she could go to Arizona. Yes, she could take whoever wished to go with her. Yes, he would give them all an official obedience and his blessing. There was no need to delay. The sooner the better. For everyone. The April council minutes record

...the obedience asked and obtained by Mother Stanislaus, March 1883 and by her two Sisters, Sr. F. Joseph and Sr. Josephine, April 10, 1883, for leaving the diocese with the intention of founding elsewhere another community under the direction of Mother Stanislaus.[3]

The three Leary sisters were joined by Sister Joseph

Teresa (who did not return to her family after all) and the four set out on their great adventure. At Nazareth there was a tearful good-bye. This was a very real ending. Things would never be the same.

New missionaries: a certain symmetry

Twenty-nine years before, four Sisters had left Carondelet and come east to Canandaigua, not knowing what they would find; now four others directly "descended" from them, boarded a train bound for an unknown western territory. There was a certain symmetry to it.

The Rochester community had in some ways lost its original missionary spirit when it agreed to be the diocesan teaching congregation. That decision anchored them, gave them security, even privilege, but it necessarily concentrated their vision. This total absorption in the one ministry of Catholic schools confirmed them as excellent, sought-after teachers and this reputation grew. However, it allowed little creativity or freedom to explore other needs or other locations. They were in Rochester to stay.

Many of the Sisters who stayed would long remember Mother Stanislaus' leaving, with sadness at losing her and regret for not having packed up to join her. These four were the missionaries now, as surely as Mother Agnes Spencer's little group had been in 1854.

Ann Leary said good-bye to her three strapping girls, pale and nervous from the events of the past months. Their community, at once grieved and relieved, was torn deeply apart.

When the little group finally settled in their new mission they would be well-equipped to do what they did best--teach-- but they brought more than skill. They had a new spirit, a new freedom, a fresh start. The journey itself was a study in freedom. Though the train ride to Kansas

City was uneventful (in sharp contrast to the snow-driven misery of the Spencer journey three decades before), their real future began with a change of plans. In Chicago they bought tickets for Kansas. From there they would make final plans for the long journey ahead of them to the far Arizona Territory.

Mother Stanislaus wrote in her diary that when they arrived in Kansas City they heard of dangerous confrontations between the settlers and the Indians in Arizona. They were too frightened to go on: four inexperienced, unaccompanied women from the urban East, completely on their own, forbidden from contacting the community in Rochester, far from family or friends who might help them.[4] They stood poised on the outer edge of the world they knew.

Bishop Louis Fink had repeatedly requested Sisters for his large diocese, which encompassed all of Kansas. Mother Stanislaus contacted him, accepted his offer, changed all their plans and headed for Leavenworth, ready for an assignment.

The "Weeding of the Garden"

All of this mind-changing would have thoroughly annoyed Bishop McQuaid who was having problems of his own with the locals. The Rochester community went through the motions of ending the school year, of holding to the familiar routines, of acting as though things had not utterly changed for them.

Sister Armella informed the council that she was leaving to join Mother Stanislaus. They ignored her. As soon as the superior at St. Patrick's left for retreat, she simply left the house and the community, without benefit of official permission, bishop's obedience or fond farewell. She had planned to go straight to Kansas, but Bishop

McQuaid made her wait two months for her papers as punishment for her unorthodox departure.[5]

Sister Antonius decided that she could not make her vows and left at the end of July, intending to go to Kansas. She never made it, but Sister Antoinette Cuff did, joining the group in August. In a now-decaying notebook, an unidentified young Sister recorded sketchy memories of the early days. She called this time: "The Weeding of the Garden."[6]

More Sisters than usual went to Hemlock that summer and those who were there were unaware of the intensity of the upheaval at home. They needed relaxation and healing from the draining events of the spring. Whichever side they were on, they needed rest.

Hemlock : they are not here

Hemlock really was a paradise. The big house stood on the top of a steep hill overlooking the water. Even today the lake is clean, blue, unpolluted. The wooded path to the water is steep and slippery with leaves and not for the arthritic, the asthmatic or the unsteady. The waterfront is not sandy but a narrow pebble beach cut by a lovely hillside stream. It is a gentle spot, not a majestic oceanside. The waves lap; they do not crash.

The ruins of the bishop's little house remain today. It had, at some point, burned to the ground, but one can see the layout clearly, can easily imagine him soaking in the quiet, delighting in the utter isolation of the place, walking in the vineyards, stout stick in hand for a crosier, deeply and calmly himself.

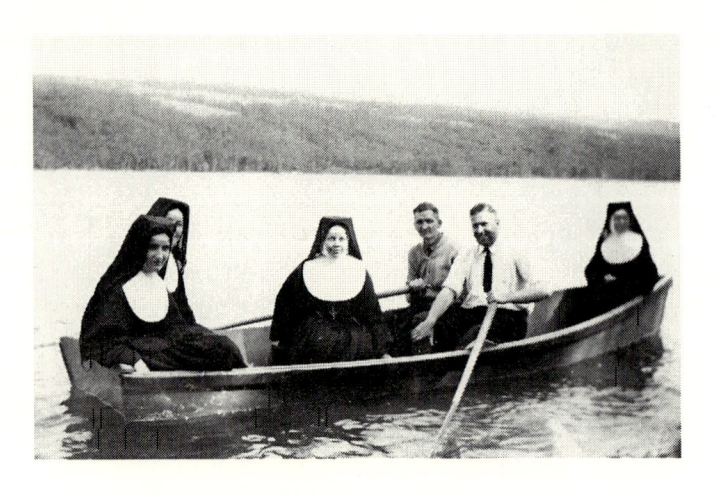

*The Sisters continued to go to Hemlock Lake,
long after the "troubles".*

And the spirits of the Sisters rest there too. Hemlock became a symbol of their closeness and their separation. Sister Berchmans had always loved the place. She used it as a metaphor for the community after so many friends left:

> When in after years some went back to revisit the old place, it did not seem the same, though it recalled to their minds other merry scenes of years gone by. The lighthearted, cheerful Sisters who caused the mirth were no longer there, and the trees, the hilltops and the lovely lake seemed sorrowfully to ask: 'Whom do you seek? They are not here.'[7]

Transplanted to Kansas: no turning back

Bishop Fink was delighted with the unexpected arrival of Sisters of St. Joseph to Kansas (more by default than by design, but the result was the same). He sent them at once to Newton to work under the blunt, rough, ardent, angry Rev. Felix Swemberg, an early advocate for Catholic colonization in Kansas.[8] Swemberg was not used to having women about, nor of having his orders questioned. But he wanted a school.

Felix Swemberg and Mother Stanislaus were very guarded with each other from the start. She had come too far to be mistreated by another controlling priest. This time she would not begin from a subservient position.

In the 1870s Newton had had a reputation as "one of the wildest towns of the western frontier." Settlers had problems with gamblers, cowboys and the "soiled doves" of the dance halls.[9] By the mid 80s, when the Sisters arrived, Newton had a Santa Fe railroad depot, a drug store, an opera house and a jail--sure signs of domestication. Many townspeople were themselves transplanted Easterners. They were ready for the brand of education offered by the New York Sisters, with its emphasis on the arts, languages and moral training.

There is no evidence that the citizens of Newton had been influenced by the strong fundamentalist preachers who lived to rid the new West of "Catholics, Mormons and moral decay."[10] When the Sisters opened their select and parochial schools on October, only about half of the students were Catholic.

But it was not an easy beginning.

They made it through a summer of real poverty. They had been used to some degree of comfort in Rochester: good furniture, tasteful Victorian ambiance at the motherhouse, adequate, nourishing food. They had lived simply, but not in poverty. It was obvious that they had little idea of what life in the frontier would be like. They had no real source of income and so were dependent on the will of the disagreeable Fr. Swemberg. Mother Stanislaus wrote in her diary:

We suffered much from poverty till the school opened...the necessaries of life we often needed. our beds were poor straw pallets, our pillows shavings and straw. The priest, Rev. Father Swemberg, had shown marked unkindness to us...One act of kindness from him we have not received...In our isolated and unprotected position we feel this very much.[11]

Whatever else Bernard McQuaid was, he was usually a gentleman. However stern and autocratic he could be, he had his gentler side and he was certainly attentive to the needs of the women he so needed to do the work in his diocesan schools. Had they made a terrible mistake in coming here? They began to have second thoughts about the whole venture.

"We often became discouraged enough," wrote Mother Stanislaus, "to break up the mission; but when we considered the wants of the poor children here and how much they would lose, we cheered up and continued."[12]

It was also, of course, a matter of pride. They had left Rochester; in effect, they had broken off from Rochester. Perhaps they had acted rashly, but it was too late now to replay the decision. They could not return, failures, begging to be readmitted. There was really no turning back for them.

It was all too much for Sister Joseph Teresa. She had a breakdown in August (she "lost her mind" is how Mother Stanislaus put it)[13]. Mother Stanislaus took her to St. Louis, to a mental hospital run by the Sisters of Charity. After she was released, Mother Stanislaus would not receive her back to the community. This was no place for the emotionally fragile.

In the fall they opened their two schools--a select boarding school and St. Mary's Parochial School. Now they were in their element. They would have an independent income and could remove themselves from the pastor's uncomfortable control.

That winter Mother Stanislaus suffered painfully from the old lung condition that had dogged her since childhood. She was so ill that the others began to ask what they would do if anything happened to her. She was the soul of this mission, the glue that held them together. Without her, could they go on?

Swemberg complained about them to Bishop Fink. Fink appointed Franciscan, Father Dominic Meier, to investigate the group. On April 26, 1884 Meier wrote to McQuaid:

> Rt. Rev. and Dear Sir!
> Would your Lordship please give me some information concerning certain Sisters of St. Joseph? Some few months ago Sisters of St. Joseph from Rochester, New York were received by our Rt. Rev. Bishop L.M. Fink and established themselves at Newton, Kansas. There are at present five in number and Ven. Sr. Stanislaus is the Mother. Shortly after their arrival they got into trouble with their Pastor, Rev. Father Swemberg and this has continued until the present day. Now our Rt. Rev. Bishop appointed me as their Superior and to investigate into their affairs. I would consider it a great favor if your Lordship would please let me know whether they left the Motherhouse with the required faculties and permission? I have been warned they were persons who could not agree with the Ven. Mother Agnes and therefore they left with the intentions of establishing a house of their own.
> Any information your Lordship will give me will be accepted with the greatest thanks! Yours in Xt,
> Rev. Dominic Meier O.S.F.[14]

By this time the group consisted of the Learys, Armella and Antoinette. Sister Domitilla joined them soon, but they were still a tiny splinter group, not a force to be dealt with.

McQuaid must have reassured Father Dominic, because there is no evidence of further investigation. It was to his advantage to keep them in Kansas. He still kept his ban on communication with the "defectors." Each month he brought it up to the council, and urged stronger vigilance among those who might still be writing or receiving letters from Kansas. Homesick, Mother Stanislaus, wrote to him in May, begging permission to keep in contact with her Sisters in Rochester:

> Ever respected Bishop--I know you will think it presumptuous in me to address you by letter now; still I will set aside all such considerations in the hope that you will grant my prayer. Will you allow me to correspond at times with my dear community of Rochester? I promise you, Right Reverend Bishop, that there will be nothing in this correspondence objectionable. I have no desire but that you should examine my letters before delivering them if such is your good pleasure.[15]

This is the last extant correspondence between them. If he answered at all, he surely refused her request. In August he made his position on the subject perfectly clear. The council minutes report:

> His Lordship again recommends prudence and wisdom in our intercourse with priests and forbids communication with those who have deserted our community. He remarks that his former orders concerning this have not been strictly obeyed.[16]

He chose to treat Mother Stanislaus and her followers as he had James Early, as he did anyone who he felt had betrayed or defied him - with silence. His attention remained in Rochester, remained with the reborn community. He truly seemed to have believed that the first fourteen years, having gone sour for him, were a closed book and that this was a renaissance.

New life in Rochester : their memory is erased

1884 was a perfect year for a renaissance: the fiftieth anniversary of the City of Rochester. Bishop McQuaid found a prime piece of property for the community to buy: a seventy acre farm on Lake Avenue. Besides being a great investment (if it became necessary, they could sell it off parcel by parcel), they could use the three buildings for their ministries and realize some money to help pay the considerable debts on the Jay Street property.

They immediately opened a private school for boys, Nazareth Hall. The bishop allowed this even though he preferred that Catholic children attend parochial schools. Nazareth Hall would be an independent source of income, as the Academy had been. Eventually this property would also be the site of his dream, a normal school for parochial school teachers. His work force would be home-grown and consistently trained.

The dissenters were hundreds of miles away, making their way on the frontier. The split was final. Once they knew that there would be no more contact with Rochester, that the door was really closed, they began a renaissance of their own.

Today, you can see the difference from the air.

As soon as you cross the Mississippi River, leave the sprawl of Kansas City and head west, the cloudless sky lets you see the amazing expanse of flat, checkerboard farmland, dots of small communities, surprise of cities.

The prairie is a state of mind. A strong sense of place: planted, rooted, wed to the land. A far horizon: uncluttered sight lines, open and ready, vulnerable to sun and storm,

I tried to see it all as she might have, a stranger

from the urban East. My first quick thought was "There's nowhere to hide here."

The Kansas they came to was a mix of transplanted gentility and rugged frontier. The terrain could not have been more different from Upstate New York. Their lives were changed, utterly.

They would not speak of their former life. Always, in years to come, when curious "descendants" in the community would urge older members to recall those days, to piece together their beginnings, they would ask: What happened in Rochester? Why did they come here?

And the answer would invariably be: "No one ever talked about it."

12 WHAT THE PAST HAS MADE US

We are what the past has made us...The perishable emotions and the momentary acts of bygone years are the scaffolding on which we build up the being that we are.

Mother Stanislaus *Diary*, January 2, 1889

In 1884 the United States bishops, in the 3rd Plenary Council of Baltimore, named Catholic schools as a top pastoral priority. There was more interest than ever in the work these Sisters could do, a growing need for schools and experienced teachers.

In Kansas there was special interest in private academies as well. In many of the small communities in the new West, public education stopped with eighth grade. Families who wanted college education for their children needed secondary schools to fill the gap. Church-related academies and prep schools sprung up throughout the West.[1]

Schools were what these Sisters did best. Mother Stanislaus had displeased McQuaid when she accepted Father O'Brien's request to staff Houses of Protection in Massachusetts. She had wanted to diversify their ministries then; now she saw that the future of her community depended on their commitment to Catholic schools.

Ironically, she had Bernard McQuaid to thank for assuring their success in the western missions. His insistence on excellence in pedagogy, in thoroughness of teacher preparation, in strictness of religious observance, painful as it eventually became, had toughened them, had given them a security that they needed to endure and increase.

They stopped looking back. The painful Rochester years became dimmer as the work widened, their numbers increased and the West opened up. Before Mother Stanislaus was through, her community would have established thirty-one missions in eight states. Her life would never be without controversy.

In spite of McQuaid's ban, she continued to have New York contacts: Julia Perry, a Nazareth Academy graduate, a talented musician, became the first postulant in the Kansas foundation; Fathers James Early, William Morrin and James Leary corresponded with her and encouraged her in her new life; Buffalo Bishop Stephen Ryan remained a quiet support; Thomas McGrath, a wealthy businessman from Niagara Falls, New York, kept an eye on the new mission. And (shades of Alice Seymour!) there was "Baroness" deZeng.

The "Baroness" deZeng: a quirky connection to the East

Mary deZeng belonged to a wealthy Episcopalian family in Geneva, New York. She had converted to Catholicism in middle age and evidently had known Mother Stanislaus through Father Morrin. When she discovered that Mother Stanislaus had abruptly left Rochester, she sent off a passionate letter telling of her distress, expressing her bitterness at the treatment Mother Stanislaus had received, blaming it all on an unnamed priest who was pastor in Geneva. "Rev. Father _____ is so queer," she wrote, " and I shall always feel that he is at the bottom of all this that Bishop M_____ has done. He is so determined and so severe...I have never felt but the one feeling for him--FEAR."[2]

She was confident that Bishop McQuaid admired Mother Stanislaus and that all the trouble would pass over in time. "I long to hear from you on what will the Bishop do next or where he will let you go, " she continued. " I'm sure the plain truth is he appreciates you too much to let any other diocese possess you."[3]

Mary deZeng seems to have been alone in her assessment. She was devoted to Mother Stanislaus. She signs this letter "Your attached friend" and says, "If Our Dear Lord will only permit me to be near you in your life I ask for no deeper joy." She could not imagine that the bishop did not share her admiration. Mother Stanislaus' reply does not survive, but she must have made it clear that this was not a temporary visit to Kansas, that she was not coming back.

Mary deZeng was a woman of means, of a prominent Geneva family. Her father, a descendant of Saxon nobility, was named after the Baron von Steuben, and Mother Stanislaus referred to her as "Baroness deZeng," a polite misnomer. Family and friends were far from overjoyed when Mary turned "Papist" and she felt alone and confused. Mistaking her new-found piety for a religious vocation, with a convert's zeal and mid-life angst she boarded a train for Newton, Kansas.

Like Alice Seymour at Nazareth, Mary deZeng lasted only a few months among the Sisters. Her presence had irritated the grumpy Father Swemberg. He complained to Bishop Fink, not wanting to deal with the Sisters directly. The bishop questioned Mother Stanislaus: Who was this woman? What was she doing with the Sisters? Who was paying for her room and board?

Mother Stanislaus wrote, assuring him that Mary deZeng was a guest and not a burden on parish finances:

> The Baroness deZeng, that has been visiting me, is not a member of our community. Hers was a visit of friendship and not as a postulant. She is in poor health and sixty years old...If I had any idea that Rev. Father did not want so many here, I would have written to you on this subject before. So far we have not been to him or the parish any extra expense.[4]

Within a year the "Baroness" was back in Geneva. In spite of her declaration to the bishop, Mother Stanislaus had indeed considered Mary deZeng a postulant. In 1884 she noted in her diary: "Miss deZeng of Geneva, N.Y. entered as a postulant but showed a decided want of vocation and returned home."[5] She must have found it necessary to bend the truth if they were to retain any independence from priests and people.

Concordia

In the fall of 1884 the Sisters opened a school in Concordia, a small town settled for fewer than twenty-five years. By the next spring they had begun an academy, and received postulants into the community. The house in Concordia became the new motherhouse.

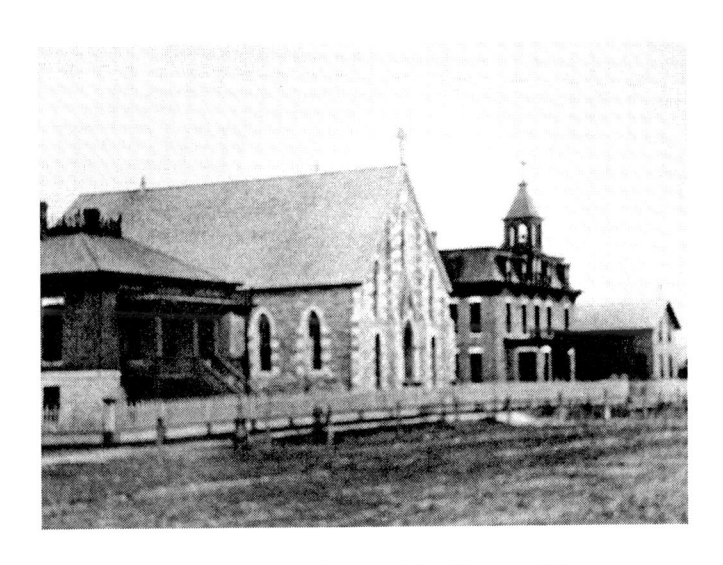

The first motherhouse of the Sisters of St. Joseph in Concordia, Kansas. This house is still in use today as a retreat center, Manna House.

Kansas was exploding with settlers. One diocese was no longer enough for the growing Catholic population. Two years later the diocese split. Concordia became a separate diocese, with Richard Scannell as its first bishop. Mother Stanislaus, wary of bishops, had feared that they might have some difficulty if an unsympathetic bishop were appointed, but the Concordia community felt comfortable at once with Bishop Scannell.

Because this was real mission territory, many women were attracted to the work, not only from Kansas and neighboring states, but from Pennsylvania, New York, Canada, France, Germany and Scotland. Margaret Leary never lost her touch, her ability to attract and hold loyalties.

The Sisters made trips to the East, in search of financial support and new candidates. Community records mention travel expenses to Buffalo and Erie (Rochester would have been out of the question!). In 1885 Mother

Stanislaus visited Erie (her old friend Agnes Spencer's foundation). A young Sister, Bernard Sheridan, was so impressed by Mother Stanislaus' enthusiastic descriptions of their work in the mysterious western missions that she left Erie to join the Concordia group.

The illness that had plagued Mother Stanislaus for so many years, and which had caused so much anxiety for the group during their first months in Kansas, never quite left her. Sister Bernard acted as her personal nurse and they became close friends. This initial closeness made the rift that would come even more bitter. Abilene would be the center of a new controversy.

Abilene had been famous as a cow town on the Chisholm Trail. By the mid-eighties the long cattle drives were over and the settlers, rid at last of troublesome cowboys, were proud of their modern and progressive town. An 1887 promotional pamphlet describes Abilene as a place settled by mostly Eastern-born people who were:

unusually intelligent as a class...clean macadamized streets, broad and beautifully graded avenues, along which are builded [sic] the largest number, proportionately, of modern city residences that grace east or west...and streets brilliantly illuminated with Edison's incandescent electric light and makes the night cheerful as the day."[6]

The same pamphlet mentions that "a young ladies" college is in the course of construction under the management and auspices of the Sisters of St. Joseph Society..."[7]

Bishop Fink had asked the Concordia community to take on an academy in Abilene, though it was in his, not in Bishop Scannell's, jurisdiction. Mother Stanislaus agreed to take it on. She took great pains to be sure that the Abilene house was well furnished and had a comfortable ambiance.

Years later Sister Madeline Perry would explain the

special care and outlay of money for the Abilene house: Mother Stanislaus presumed that Kansas would be further divided into new dioceses. If she did not like whoever took Bishop Scannell's place in Concordia, she would simply move the motherhouse to Abilene, where her friend Bishop Fink had jurisdiction. She would take no chances with bishops.[8]

Bishop Fink was thinking along the same lines. He wanted to be sure to retain the Sisters of St. Joseph in his diocese and even asked Mother Stanislaus to come to Abilene then, to be the superior of the new group, to start receiving candidates there - in effect, to switch their headquarters from Concordia to Abilene.

A split, a piano, and wounds that wouldn't heal

As usual, the tug-of-war and the ultimate decision was between the bishops, not among the Sisters. At least, not at first. Bishop Scannell would not hear of their moving to another diocese. Bishop Fink wanted them in his. The only solution was a split. Mother Stanislaus must have been taken back to 1868, when Bishop McQuaid had given their Buffalo community the same choice: go back to Buffalo or start a new foundation with me. Only, this time she was on the other side.

Sisters Bernard, Domitilla, Armella and Sebastian opted to stay in Abilene and establish a new motherhouse there. If it felt familiar to Mother Stanislaus in one way, this parting, this dividing of a young community was different from the one she had experienced in Buffalo twenty-one years before. This division was charged with the pain of close friends who can no longer talk to each other, who cannot reach beyond a disagreement to find what was at the core of their separation.

Mother Stanislaus had had a special bond with

Armella and Domitilla. They had literally given up everything to follow her to Kansas. They had all been pioneers together, had shared the hard beginnings, had held on to the hope and excitement of creating something risky and new. Bernard, too, was only there because of her. They had grown close in the four short years they had known each other, and Mother Stanislaus had shown her confidence in Sister Bernard by making her superior of the Abilene community.

Was she devastated by the eagerness they seemed to have for independence? Did she see this as a personal betrayal? Whatever the motivation, Mother Stanislaus' reaction now seems both petty and punitive. The bishops drew up the required papers for the division of the community and the transfer of deeds. Mother Stanislaus went to Abilene to sign the papers. The meeting seemed amiable enough, but after she returned to Concordia she sent word to the Abilene group that they would have to return the furniture from the house, including the handsome square piano, or reimburse the Concordia community for it.

She characterized it as a matter of justice; it was obviously something else. There is even evidence that she (or someone) doctored the account book, inflating the prices for the furniture, piano and other costs at the Abilene house.[9] If there remained any of the old loyalty, any shred of past friendship, this disturbing demand seems to have ended it. The Abilene community simply ignored her demand and with that came a rift that was so complete that for years newer members of the community never even knew that Mother Bernard Sheridan had ever been in Concordia at all.[10]

Eventually, a second division of dioceses in Kansas placed Mother Bernard's community in the Wichita diocese and they established their motherhouse in that growing river city.

Mother Stanislaus kept a sporadic diary, a combination of recorded events, spiritual "gems" copied from other sources, poetry, even recipes. Entries she made at the start of 1889 reveal her state of mind as she dealt with the realities of the community split:

> As the tree is fertilized by its own broken branches and fallen leaves and grows out of its own decay, so is the soul refined out of broken hopes and blighted affections.

> We are what the past has made us...The perishable emotions and the momentary acts of bygone years are the scaffolding on which we build up the being that we are.

And was she thinking of her lost friends when she wrote:

> May all go well with you, may life's short day glide on, peaceful and bright with no more clouds than may glisten in the sunshine and no more rain than may form a rainbow; and may the veiled one of heaven bring us to meet again.[11]

Slammming the door to the past

Later that year she recorded that she suffered from heart trouble (cause or effect of her uncharacteristic toughness with the Abilene group?); then a terse, cryptic note: "Crosses and trials..."[12]

One of the crosses was the death of her sister Isabelle in Rochester. Isabelle was the "Mrs. Matthews" at whose home she and Father Early had met to avoid the scrutiny of Bishop McQuaid on her return from Florida. Not many months later she would hear of James Early's death as well.

From the time he left the Rochester diocese in 1876, James Early had continued to plague Bishop McQuaid with his stubborn (almost frivolous) law suit. After Mother Stanislaus' removal, he had heated up the fight even more.

He had irritated McQuaid by coming to Rochester from Hornellsville to gain supporters for his cause. His boldness infuriated the bishop. The lion did not care to be bearded in his own den. Now Early was dying of a slow degenerative disease. McQuaid knew it, but he never could bring himself to offer a word of friendship or comfort to his one-time friend.

James Early died on February 17, 1890 and on February 18 his friend Father Peter Colgan from neighboring Corning, wrote McQuaid:

I want to let you know that Father Early expressed a great desire to see you before he died. He said he was quick and so were you but would like very much to see you...With regard to the amount of money in dispute between himself and you, that is all settled. You will get no more trouble on that score. I would like very much and I think it would look very nice if you would come to his funeral. It would give great edification to priests and people...[13]

McQuaid must not have replied to this letter, and did not attend the funeral, despite Father Colgan's mentioning that it would "look very nice" if he did. After the funeral, he wrote the bishop again, to clarify the settlement of the lawsuit:

With regard to Fr. Early's affair, the Friday before he died, he expressed a great desire to see you. I blamed Sr. Catharine [sic][14] for not sending you a dispatch at once...Catharine did not think he would die so soon. He wrote a note which is in Sister Catharine's care yet, and this is the substance, that the judgment for $8000 against the trustees of St. Patrick's Cathedral Rochester be cancelled.[15]

Early had had no intention, evidently, of actually collecting from the suit. It was his only effective weapon against his old adversary. He had kept up the fight until his deathbed.

Sister Mary Catherine sent off a wire to Mother

Stanislaus: *"Father Early is dead. funeral Thursday. try to come"* [16]

If Mother Stanislaus made the journey to Hornellsville, she certainly did not visit Rochester. There is no record of any Kansas Sisters returning until Sister Josephine Leary came for Mother Agnes' Golden Jubilee in 1919. But whether or not she came to the funeral, James Early's death was surely the final slamming of the door to the past for her.

13 THE DUST FROM MY FEET

> *I remember Mother Stanislaus came into the Novitiate just as much as to say 'Well, I am not accountable for this. I shake the dust from under my feet.'* Those were her last words to the Novices.
>
> Sister Evelyn Fraser, CSJ Concordia

As early as 1897 Mother Stanislaus had sent out feelers to Mother Clement of Chestnut Hill, Pennsylvania, asking about the possibility and the process for uniting the Concordia community with theirs. Mother Clement had sent, at Mother Stanislaus' request, copies of their Rule and Customs book, and invited Concordia's Mistress of Novices to stay with the Chestnut Hill community for a time.[1]

Mother Stanislaus asked for complete secrecy about the reason for these exchanges and evidently no one in Concordia questioned this new closeness with a faraway community. They didn't know she was considering a merger. Her authority and control over the community seem to have been absolute. With no bishop to question her right to make such decisions, she assumed supreme authority with a truly McQuaid-like autocracy.

Money problems were weighing her down; she was in constant pain; she was emotionally fragile. She was enough of a realist to know that she would not be capable to lead the community much longer. Perhaps she thought its only chance for survival was as a missionary branch of an older, well-established congregation of the Sisters of St. Joseph. In February 1898, still begging for secrecy, she offered to send a novice to be trained at Chestnut Hill, as a sort of test case, a prelude to their eventual union.

Mother Clement was growing apprehensive about the proposal. She wrote worried letters to a friend, Father Sabetti, who told her bluntly that she should stop these negotiations and tell Mother Stanislaus that such a union of communities was not an option.[2] Concordia would have to make it on its own.

John Cunningham was officially installed as Bishop of Concordia on September 21, 1898, ending Mother Stanislaus' unusual term as final authority. In November Mother Stanislaus visited some out-of-state missions in Wisconsin, Michigan and northern Illinois. Her health began to break down seriously during that trip. A nerve disease was causing her untold pain and a rough carriage ride on muddy, rutted roads had turned her spine into a mass of bruises. Her hands and feet gave her great pain. On her return to Kansas, she fainted dead away at the Clyde train depot. Concordia doctors could not help her, and suggested that she try mineral baths in Excelsior Springs, Arkansas.

Sister Alexine Gosslein became her companion, nurse and confidant in the painful months ahead. Though she gave the impression of utter self sufficiency, Mother Stanislaus seems always to have needed the undivided attention of one other person when she was in trouble:

Baptista Hanson, her mentor through the puzzling Rochester years, had earned McQuaid's wrath by encouraging Mother Stanislaus to claim her own authority; Ursula Murphy had put her own life on hold to become her companion in her Florida exile; Bernard Sheridan had been her personal nurse when sickness threatened her ability to lead the young Concordia community; now, Alexine became her nurse-cum-confidant. The others had paid a price for their friendship with her. So would Alexine.

She tried the mineral baths. They gave no relief. They went to Chicago to see a specialist; from there to a sanitarium in Lake Geneva, Wisconsin; then back to Chicago. The doctor wanted her to stay in the Chicago area so they could observe her and try to treat her baffling condition.

Months passed. Mother Stanislaus had become an absentee superior of the Concordia community. It appears that there was little or no contact with her Sisters in Kansas during this time. They must have wondered what she was up to. Concordia's missions were so far-flung. Was she looking in Chicago for a more central place for their headquarters? Was she planning, even then, to begin an entirely new foundation? Why wasn't there a stream of letters between Chicago and Concordia? There was only silence.

In Chicago, Father Martell, the pastor of St. John Baptist Church, contacted Mother Stanislaus: Would her Concordia Sisters consider staffing his parish school? These Sisters had a great reputation as teachers. She agreed. He offered his own house for a convent; she and Sister Alexine moved in on June 11. In Concordia they waited for word. There was only silence.

Something was going on

It was customary for the Sisters on the missions to return to Concordia for the summer. On June 30 four Sisters went to Chicago instead of going home. Sister Francis Joseph Leary, Josephine Leary, Constance Ryan and Berchmans Gray joined Mother Stanislaus and Alexine at St. John's. Something was definitely going on.
Bishop Cunningham sent for Mother Stanislaus in early July. What happened next can only be pieced together, a patchwork of hearsay, sketchy records, community tradition, and the coaxed-out memories of two eyewitnesses.
Sister Isabelle Poisson was a young Sister in 1899. In 1975 she taped her recollections of those days. She recalled that it was generally accepted in the community at the time that "they asked the bishop for a change." When asked who "they" were, she said, "The officers who were in charge at the time."[3]
There was some problem with community funds, a "misunderstanding about expenditures," Sister Isabelle remembered. Then, quick to defend Mother Stanislaus, she tried to explain:

(Mother Stanislaus) didn't intend to do anything, only she was in hard circumstances. The mission was just beginning and there were so many places to be looked after and not much money coming in and there were difficulties. She was helping poor people too, and maybe that caused trouble...[4]

There had been some irregularities in bookkeeping. The pattern was familiar. In Rochester, James O'Hare had stripped Mother Stanislaus of any power over or contact with St. Mary's Asylum because of some unauthorized loans. Her bookkeeping practices had been "creative" at Nazareth Convent--not necessarily illegal, but certainly robbing Peter to pay Paul.[5] Evidently, she had been at it again in Concordia. When the financial situation was made public in the community, Mother Stanislaus was crushed, humiliated. She became sick.[6]

Since young Sisters were rarely privy to the workings of those in office, it is hard to tell how much of this second-hand testimony is valid and how much community lore. There was no attempt to tell all the Sisters what the real situation was. Sister Isabelle recalled: "It was all done privately...We didn't discuss personalities...all we had to do was obey the rules and follow up...It was all done privately."[7]

It all came to a head in July 1899. Mother Stanislaus must have finally returned to Concordia, at least for a time. She was there when the new bishop sent for Sister Antoinette Cuff, gathered the Sisters in the motherhouse chapel and announced Antoinette's appointment as Superior General.

Angry, bewildered, deeply hurt, Mother Stanislaus left the chapel alone. Leaning heavily on the railing, she climbed the stairs one slow step at a time. Upstairs she heard someone greet her, with peculiar venom, as "Sister Stanislaus." Since even local superiors were given the honorary title of "Mother," calling her "Sister" cruelly rubbed salt in a very fresh wound. She felt herself becoming a stranger here, as she had in Rochester. Sister Isabelle remembered:

No one could do anything for her...We didn't see much of her anymore after that...she must have gotten ready right away and left the next day...'It is gone! No hope,' she said...We didn't get to see her, but we all felt badly. Some of them said, 'Oh, I'm ready to go home,' but they didn't go.[8]

Sister Evelyn Fraser had been a novice at the time.

She clearly recalled the day Mother Antoinette's appointment was announced:

I remember Mother Stanislaus came to the Novitiate just as much as to say 'Well, I am not accountable for this. I shake the dust from under my feet.' Those were her last words to the Novices...We were kind of stunned, you know. We didn't know anything about what was happening.[9]

These are memories recalled well over seventy years after they took place. If the details are fuzzy or the quotes imprecise, there is no mistaking the emotion that these women still felt in thinking of Mother Stanislaus' leaving.

It had been the same in Rochester. An old story describes the Sisters at Nazareth clinging to the carriage wheels, trying to stop her from leaving for the train station.[10] Even if the story is apocryphal, the recollected emotion, the frustration and sorrow of the Sisters are clear.

Bishop Cunningham was no Bernard McQuaid. He had no personal quarrel with Mother Stanislaus; they had no bitter history. His removal of Mother Stanislaus was neither the result of a contest of wills nor a desire to retain control of a religious congregation. He had made the change on the advice of a former bishop and members of the congregation. He bore her no ill will. Still, the abruptness of the change, the reality of stepping down, the seeming indifference of some of the members of the community, and her own failing health made her next step clearer. She could not stay in Concordia. At least not for now.

She returned to St. John's where the group was making plans to open the school in September. After a few weeks of cooling-off, she returned to Concordia to finalize the transfer of office and to talk with the Bishop. She had a new agenda. Chicago Archbishop Patrick Feehan was interested in having the Sisters of St. Joseph in his diocese. Mother Stanislaus requested an official obedience from Bishop Cunningham to allow her and the others to stay in Chicago. He refused. She returned to Chicago, shaken by the refusal. Sister Alexine, hovering and concerned, was alarmed by her appearance. Clearly she was weaker; she needed rest, not a new fight.

In Concordia there was a rumor of some irregularity in the Chicago house. There was even talk of a split, of a secret plan to start a new foundation there. Mother Antoinette sent Sister Mary Ann Picard and two others to St. John's to see what was going on, and to take charge of the new school. They arrived at the convent door unannounced, flatly stating that the mission at St. John's had been entrusted to their hands. The encounter must have been high drama.

Sister Alexine was in the drug store, having a prescription filled for Mother Stanislaus. Someone ran in to tell her that some strange Sisters were at the house and she was to return quickly. By the time she got home, Mother Stanislaus had already decided that they would not remain in the house, that they would leave immediately. The LaGrange *Annals* simply state:

She lost no time in ordering a conveyance to take the Sisters and their belongings from St. John's and in the course of a few hours Rev. Mother Stanislaus and her faithful daughters were winding their way through the great city, not knowing where to go.[11]

They had no money, no destination. They were literally homeless. Mother Stanislaus' decision to pack up and leave seems rash and unnecessary, even irrational, but the unexpected arrival of the Concordia Sisters had hurt and angered her and she had reacted out of those strong emotions. The others had blindly followed her lead. Now, here they were, riding around Chicago, nursing their bruised pride, their dignity intact but their home gone.

The six put their heads together as calmly as they could as they rode around Chicago in that cab. One look at Mother Stanislaus told them that she was near collapse. They decided that she needed to go to a hospital at once. Sister Constance would go with her, and the others would ask the Good Shepherd Sisters to take them in temporarily.

It was while she was in the hospital that Mother Stanislaus began negotiations with Archbishop Feehan to start a separate foundation in the Chicago Archdiocese. It has never been clear how far these arrangements got while she was still alive, but she promised to begin an academy in the diocese as soon as they could. They still did not have official permission to leave Concordia. They had no independent status. They really belonged nowhere.

Thomas McGrath, Mother Stanislaus' wealthy friend in Niagara Falls, was also a friend of Father James Hagan, the pastor in LaGrange, a prosperous Chicago suburb. On McGrath's recommendation, Father Hagan invited the Sisters to come to LaGrange.

On October 2, 1899 they rented a house in LaGrange, but found they couldn't afford to stay. They moved afterwards to a smaller place on Spring Avenue, near the church. It was clear that in spite of his invitation, Father Hagan had no intention of supporting the group or of giving them an active role in the parish. They were badly in need of money, and had even taken to begging for food among the people. This did not endear them to the pastor.

Mother Stanislaus came home from the hospital in November, but she was failing rapidly. She had directed the acceptance of a young Sister, Sister Ligouri (who seems to have been in another St. Joseph community and joined them as a novice) and a widow as a postulant.

It has never been clear whether Mother Stanislaus intended to stay in Chicago when she left Concordia, whether she had intended to begin a new foundation. No longer the Superior General of the Concordia community, she actually had no authority to open new houses and establish new missions in the name of Concordia. Such decisions, after so many years, must have been second nature to her. Perhaps she did not think of them as the acts of the superior of a separate group. She was unused to asking someone else's permission to act. There is no evidence that she consulted Mother Antoinette about these decisions. When she began accepting new members, it was clearly as a person with authority separate from Concordia.

Her physical condition was serious; she was weak, sleepless and in constant pain. In some ways, her heart was in Kansas still. Later, they would hear in Concordia that when Mother Stanislaus was dying, she had cried out: "Where am I? I don't belong here. I belong in Concordia. I want to die in Concordia with my own."[12]

Burning bridges once more

But once again she had burned her bridges. There was no returning to Concordia any more than there could have been a return to Rochester. Alexine was totally devoted to her. She slept at the foot of Mother Stanislaus' bed, talking with her if she were wakeful, feeding her when she could eat, wrapping her hands and feet with ice and towels to relieve the pain.

Mother Stanislaus had one more thing to do: she had made a commitment to Archbishop Feehan. She selected a site for an academy and motherhouse and name a reluctant Sister Alexine as her choice for superior of the new group. Sisters Josephine and Francis Joseph, though they fully appreciated Alexine's devotion, did not take kindly to this clear favoritism. But this was not the time for jealousy or personal enmity. They knew that their sister was desperately sick, and they put their wounded feelings on hold.

To the day she died Alexine herself held that she never meant to leave Concordia and certainly did not see herself as a leader. But she knew it did no good to argue with Mother Stanislaus when she talked this way. She decided to humor her. She promised to carry on the work.

Christmas of 1899 came and went and the nineteenth century turned to the twentieth with a worldwide New Years celebration.

14 IN A BORROWED GRAVE

> *This earthy life has been fitly characterized as a pilgrimage through a valley of tears. Everything in this world is characterized by imperfection. The best people have many faults. The clearest mind only sees through a glass darkly, the purest heart is not without spot. We cannot wholly trust either ourselves or our fellow men.*
>
> *Every heart has its grief, every house has its skeleton, every character is marred with weakness and imperfection.*
>
> *All these aimless conflicts of our minds are unanswered longings of our hearts, and should lead us to rejoice the more in the divine mystery, the assurance that a time is coming when night shall melt into noon and the mystery shall be clothed with glory.*
>
> Mother Stanislaus Leary, *Diary*, 1896

The world of the late 1890s was a mix, as any time is a mix: prosperity and hunger, changing mores and traditional manners, progress and its bitter results.

The boll weevil crossed the Rio Grande, devastating

King Cotton. Steel, the garment industry, autos, and railroads brought exploitation, unions, violence, and reforms. Trolleys and subways buried the horsecar.

Sigmund Freud wrote *The Interpretation of Dreams;* John Dewey challenged educators with *The School and Society.* Edward Stratemeyer began his literary syndicate that would direct hack writers to grind out stories about the Bobbsey Twins, Tom Swift, the Hardy Boys, the Rover Boys and Nancy Drew.

People were singing "Because," "My Wild Irish Rose," "On the Banks of the Wabash," "The Band Played On," and "When You Were Sweet Sixteen," and dancing the cake walk as well as the waltz. Scott Joplin played ragtime and Florenz Ziegfeld became a prime purveyor of feminine beauty.

Chopped beefsteak was now called Hamburg steak, and Coca Cola, once available only at soda fountains, was sold in individual bottles.

Cezanne, G.B. Shaw, Houdini, Lillian Russell, Renoir, Puccini, William Jennings Bryant, Carry Nation, Theodore Dreiser; Kresge and Woolworth, Gilbert and Sullivan, Carnegie and Rockefeller, William Randolph Hearst and the Katzenjammer Kids; Hershey, Jell-O, Aunt Jemima, Shredded Wheat, Lipton Tea, evaporated milk, Campbell Soup, Pepsi Cola.

In Rochester, New York while George Eastman had made the Brownie camera a snap for the amateur, Bishop Bernard McQuaid had realized his dream of a strong Catholic school system and a respected major seminary. Five hundred miles away his old nemesis lay dying.

It would not be an easy dying. The doctors called her condition "rheumatism of the nerves" for want of a more specific term. They had been baffled by her symptoms: acute pain in her hands and feet; painful bruising from the smallest touch or bump. They described her nerves as "drying up from the ends." There was little done to manage her pain, and sleep eluded her.

Sister Alexine, curled up at the foot of her bed, tried to soothe her, to distract her from the pain. She remembered hearing her cry out in what she interpreted as prayer: "O Blessed Mother! O Ingratitude! O Ingratitude!"[1]

Such deathbed drama falls uncomfortably on modern ears, but there is a ring of reality in her choice of words. Tongue loosened, internal censor disregarded, honest at last, she could say the word that spoke her deepest pain: ingratitude.

Her condition worsened. Quietly, finally, in the dark night, just after one o'clock in the morning on February 14, 1900, snow falling thickly outside her window, Margaret Leary finished her long journey. Though the Kansas climate had kept her healthier than the brutal dampness of Western New York had ever done, she was still, at fifty-eight, too young to die. February 14 was the forty-third anniversary of her reception of the habit in Canandaigua. Her life, too, had had a certain symmetry.

Even in death she was the center of unrest. Deep in grief and fearful of the future, the group had to decide what to do, how and where to bury here, how to carry on without her. They had no money, no official status, no Chicago contacts other than those Mother Stanislaus herself had made.

Perhaps they approached some of her wealthy friends; perhaps they appealed to the Archbishop for help; perhaps they swallowed their pride and contacted Concordia. In any case, the decision (not a small one) was to bury her there, not to return her to Kansas. Either they got the money to pay or accepted the charity of a generous undertaker, because a photo survives of a flower-decked casket in front of an ornate wooden altar, her face waxy-perfect, still and serene as any plaster saint.

A Chicago newspaper carried an obituary the following week. It was the usual mix of fact and fiction, a life-in-capsule, a brief baedeker for her unique odyssey:

> Reverend Mother Mary Stanislaus, Superior of the Sisters of St. Joseph living on North Spring Avenue, LaGrange, died last Wednesday morning about 1 o'clock...born in New York City, August 15, 1841.
>
> In 1856 at age 15 she entered the Novitiate of the Sisters of St. Joseph in Buffalo, and spent the next eight years in that diocese...In 1864 she was sent to make a foundation in Rochester, N.Y. With four or five other Sisters she opened St. Mary's Orphan Asylum in that city; and a few years later was laid the foundation of Nazareth Convent and Academy, one of the finest educational institutions in the country...In 1882, owing to ill health, she was obliged to seek a change of climate and selected Kansas for her field of labor...At Concordia Kansas a large and flourishing community grew up under her guidance...Nearly two years ago, her health failed and, after every means of affording her relief in Kansas had been exhausted, she came to Chicago for medical treatment. However, it was too late. She had been ill for the past two months, but her illness was never regarded as serious. In fact, the doctors thought all along she would get better as she was of a rugged constitution and otherwise well preserved...
>
> She was one of the gentlest and most amiable of women and was beloved by all who knew her, especially by her spiritual daughters who have reason to mourn the loss of so devoted a Superior.[2]

It is interesting that a Chicago paper would give so much space to an obituary for someone who was not that well known in the area, who had not really done anything in the diocese, who, it seems now, had come to Illinois to die. The writer must have obtained his material totally from the little group on Spring Avenue, most probably from her own sisters who had been witnesses to all the journeys of her life and would be inclined to gloss over the harsher realities.

The Sisters of St. Joseph in Rochester heard of her

death, stirring memories long repressed among them. Years later, Sister Teresina Hayes wrote:

> The news of her death touched many hearts in the Rochester community, where her name was held in veneration by those she had trained in the spiritual life. Mother Stanislaus was endowed by nature with an amiable disposition, a childlike simplicity and an attractive personality that won all hearts. Though much of her life had been spent beneath the shadow of the cross, it was, nevertheless, a life singularly blest in its accomplishments. Two great communities in the middle west owe their origin, at least in part, to her.[3]

Discretion demanded that Sister Teresina omit the details of the "shadow of the cross" (and especially the Rochester community's part in it), but this was the first public recognition of unusual suffering in the life of the woman who had been their foundress.

She remained unburied until the spring. The ground may have been too frozen to dig a grave. Even if it had been possible to bury her, they had no plot, nor funds to buy one. Alexine was anxious to get back to Concordia; she had never meant to stay in LaGrange. She knew that the others were aware that Mother Stanislaus had named her as the leader of this new group and she knew they resented it. She would stay just long enough to bury her friend and they could all return to Kansas. Worry, fear and grief lowered her resistance and she became very ill with pneumonia.

An Irish woman in Chicago heard of the Sisters' problem and offered them a plot in Calvary Cemetery. On March 23 they took their Sister to a borrowed grave.[4]

They all knew that Mother Stanislaus had wanted this new foundation. Things had gone too far, and they had been gone too long without communicating with Concordia. Going back did not seem as certain, or even possible as it had before. Mother Stanislaus had set a few things in motion in the last months of her life, but they still did not have an obedience from Concordia's bishop, a clear word from Archbishop Feehan, or any work to do in the LaGrange parish. They were destitute, with no means of supporting themselves except begging.

Toward the end of June the Archbishop took the matter in hand. He called Alexine in and appointed her, officially, as the superior of the new community, the Sisters of St. Joseph in the Archdiocese of Chicago. This was not the news she had been hoping for. She did not want the job. Not only did it mean a final break from Concordia, and a heavy and unwelcome burden of responsibility, but (she found out when she returned home and was forced to tell the other sisters) it broke open festering wounds, jealousy, and resentment among the others.

From the moment she returned from the Episcopal residence with her new charge, Alexine had trouble. The Learys, with Sisters Constance and Berchmans behind them all the way, refused to accept her authority over them. Incredible and petty as it sounds, they formed a separate community within the same small house. They refused to associate with Alexine and the others.

Fortunately the situation didn't last long. In a few weeks, the four of them were gone, off to seek their own destinies. Evidently it had been Mother Stanislaus alone who had held that fragile group together; without her they had no center. The new community consisted of Alexine, now the Reverend Mother, a novice and a postulant. They had exactly 33¢.

Some of the people in LaGrange were suspicious of them. There were rumors that the group had rebelled against the Bishop of Concordia and struck out on their own. One woman wrote a letter to Sister Alexine a few months later calling them "runaways," having "no rule, no discipline, no honor, no honesty, no order."[5]

Mother Alexine looked for help from a priest friend

whom she trusted. Monsignor J.E. Laberge had known Mother Stanislaus, had been watching the situation as it was evolving in LaGrange. He had strong words for Alexine, honest advice and a caveat against blind hero worship:

> Do not undertake too much at once; I...think this was one of the mistakes of Mother Stanislaus. She was forced to hurry the preparation of her novices and it seems to me nothing can be more detrimental to the community that a precipitous preparation...Take much care in forming your novices...above all in the virtue of humility..
>
> .In the eyes of the people abroad, I mean those who are acquainted with the history of your community, your foundress, no doubt a pious woman, had with all her virtues the weakness of being fond of honor or at least superiority. This may be an error on the part of the public but such is the judgment. I see...that you are a great admirer of her merits; you have certainly good reasons for it, but I would advise you to eradicate from your community the least desire or aspiration on the part of your Sisters to honor or superiority.[6]

It is difficult to say how much of this advice Mother Alexine was able to take in. She was not disposed to hear criticism of someone to whom she was almost irrationally devoted. She is said to have told a group of young Sisters at LaGrange, years later, that she was personally guided by Mother Stanislaus during the first year, that she felt a palpable presence, that she asked her advice and received clear direction.[7]

It is not unusual, of course, for survivors to experience the deep presence of a loved one who has died, to feel looked after and guided by someone who had been a strong and familiar influence on them. It is no surprise that her spirit would inform the early years of this new congregation, as it had the others.

Of one thing there is no doubt: Margaret Leary was always a strong and pervading presence in her lifetime:

often a sign of division, of conflicting loyalties, of misplaced affection; often a paradox of precision and creativity, of a search for stability and love for adventure, of great kindliness and sharp authoritarianism, of calm flexibility and stubborn firmness, she struggled with humility, uneasy with domination, unable to step down with grace. Naturally the leader, the educator, the builder, the starter, she drew people to her and turned them against her with an equal force.

Even her death was ironic: penniless, virtually homeless, buried in someone else's grave, in a city she barely knew, in a kind of exile. Her new work was incomplete. The other communities she had founded were bitter fruit. They all grew without her, on their own terms, in their own ways.

The memory of those days faded. The proud beginnings were remembered, the personal conflicts hidden or glossed over, and her extraordinary life was cut to the size of a holy card.

THE REST OF THE PICTURE

As I write the last words of this story, I am again surrounded by pictures. I copied them from books, from archival prints, from periodicals; I pasted them on a board and kept them in front of me while I wrote - to help me focus, to retell the story for me, to link me to the present:

A picture I took in the 1990s of the house on Saltonstall Street in Canandaigua, as it has survived shows a wooden structure in great need of repair : the ragged roof and sagging railings looking for all the world as if they would crumble or blow away, overstuffed chairs on the upstairs porch, a battered tricycle and cast-off Big Wheels and strollers in the yard. Suspicious eyes stare flatly from curtainless window as I aim the camera, a tourist from the wrong century. The residents didn't know, no did they need to, that their home was something of a shrine.

The old Nazareth Convent on Jay Street: a strong, forbidding house, the wings and mansard roof that Mother Stanislaus added when the Bishop was in Rome, clearly visible, neatly landscaped with creative touches of shrub and tree. Almost two decades after McQuaid's death, the Motherhouse he had planned for was complete: a spacious country setting, room for administration, normal school, novitiate and infirmary. Today a public school for children with special needs stands on Old Nazareth's ground. Margaret Leary would have liked that.

St. Patrick's Cathedral and the bishop's residence: in the old pictures they look impenetrable, planned and laid brick by brick by proud Irish immigrants. Nothing lasts. Both buildings were razed in 1938, leveled, planed and paved into a parking lot for Eastman Kodak.

A picture of Bishop McQuaid, portly, top-hatted, hurrying out to the State Street trolley

A winter sketch of St. Mary's Hospital in the early 1860s: white-winged Sisters of Charity, huddled against the bitter wind, a sleigh horsecar sliding soundlessly over the hard-packed snow in front of the old inn that would become St. Mary's Boys' Asylum.

Another shot of the white-wings, sitting amid sixty or more orphan girls at St. Patrick's Asylum: they all sit straight and very still, the older girls in black frocks, bows and high button shoes, the little ones in white. Those Sisters would be leaving soon, at the bishop's direction. Others, strangers, would be taking their places. Other children would come to live their childhood in the massive brick structures the Sisters would try to make "home." In the 1940s the asylums would be combined into a spacious, cottage-based suburban campus renamed St. Joseph's Villa, now a residence for teens at risk.

In another picture, three men in cassocks stand on the porch of the Hemlock cottage. The sun is very bright, reflecting clouds and trees in the windows that ring the big house. From their vantage they can look down on steep vineyards, on the thickly-wooded path to the stony shore, on the fast-running stream that divides one from the other. All of the natural features are there to this day; a winery stands where the big house once did, and the owners sell altar wine under Bishop McQuaid's original label: O-Neh-Dah. The air is full of memories.

I stare for the hundredth time at the most puzzling picture of all, the Mystery House: seventeen Sisters of St. Joseph, in formal twos and threes, stand in front of a huge Victorian house, dwarfed by its massive stone. The architecture is eclectic: stone and slate, gingerbread trim, a deep mansard roof, turret, surrounded by orchard on a flat plain. It is an imposing rural villa. No one (no senior Sisters, no preservation experts, no local historians, no one) has seen this house.

The picture came from LeGrange, Mother Stanislaus' last foundation. Written on the back of the picture:

> *This is the home Mother Stanislaus had to give up or leave Rochester. She preferred to leave than break her word with the donors. The Sisters spent one vacation here. This place was given to Mother Stanislaus by a friend for a vacation home for the Sisters.*[1]

The Sisters are there in the picture, frozen forever in this moment. Their faces, even in enlargement, are fuzzy. I magnify them even more and compare them with old portraits of Sisters from that time--compare the tilt of head, the stance, the hand positions, the attitude of each to the camera's eye. I *think* I can see a resemblance to old pictures from that time, faces of our Sisters. But I know that I will never know.

For some reason, she kept this picture all her life. For some reason, this place, or these people, were important to her. For some reason she brought this memory with her, and not another. Its message certainly makes sense. If a benefactor had given this house to our Sisters; if Mother Stanislaus had welcomed it as an alternative to Hemlock; if Bernard McQuaid had insisted that the Congregation transfer the property to the diocese and she had refused – this would have been the final straw. It is a fact that McQuaid was looking for a place to start his seminary at that very time and there are legal papers from 1883 which state his frustration at not being able to obtain "free title" on some unnamed property.

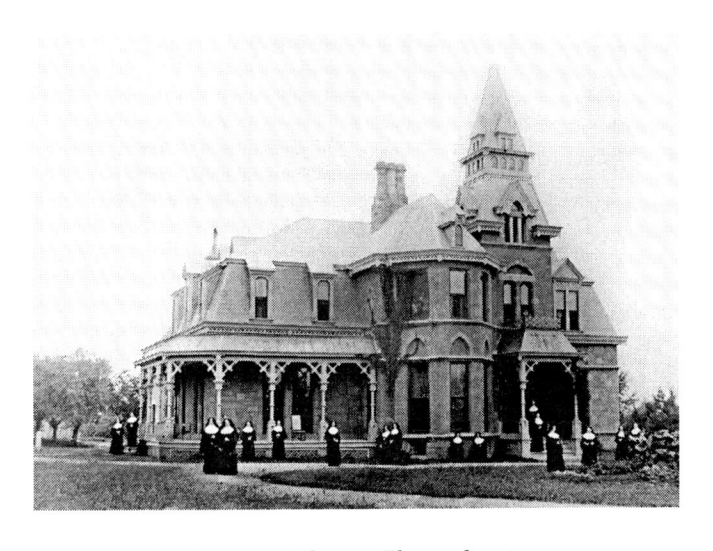

The "mystery" house. This is the picture Mother Stanislaus took with her to Kansas. No one knows exactly where the house was.

No matter what truth we think we can piece together from histories, old pictures, old papers, we can never know it all, can only look at the past through our present lenses. Facts we can know (to a degree); events we can reproduce; hearts we can only imagine. We are frozen in our own time. It's hard to lift the veil.

I look at three Kansas houses. The white clapboard in Newton, where the little Rochester group had battled Father Swemberg, received Julia Perry and the "Baroness" and spent their first hard years in Kansas. Then, the first motherhouse in Concordia: sturdy brick, roomy, standing as it does today beside the parish church. It has served as motherhouse, hospital and finally, Manna House of Prayer. The third, the house in Abelinc, its furnishings the symbol of division, of the fragility of human hearts.

186

There are portraits of the Dramatis Personae on the board as well:

Bishop John Timon, calm-faced, determined, grasps a breviary, making sure that his episcopal ring is in evidence.

Mother Agnes Spencer, sad and plain, her eyes and mouth tending downward in a stern weariness, looks older than her years.

Next to her glares her friend, the wild Irishman, Father Edmund O'Connor, mustache drooping, eyes defiant.

In the corner is a young Bishop Stephen Ryan, bespectacled, serious, mild, the opposite personality of his Rochester counterpart, B.J. McQuaid.

Mother Hieronymo O'Brien, who had had to give up the community she loved to do the work she was born for, looks out of place. She never did quite "fit," seems uncomfortable in the black habit, white linens imprisoning her face, heavy veil pinned awkwardly, giving her a look different from the others. They say she always mourned the Sisters of Charity, and loved to tell of Emmitsburg days. Today her likeness stands with a dozen or so famous Rochesterians, on permanent display at the museum of the restored historic area in Rochester. Press a button. A figure is illuminated and a tape spins a tale about Susan B. Anthony or George Eastman or Frederick Douglass or Mother Hieronymo O'Brien. No religious figure before her or since has had such an impact on the City of Rochester.

Monsignor Hippolyte DeRegge, wavy silver hair, heavy-lidded eyes and a Maurice Chevalier smile, looks straight at the photographer. In his last years he spent a good deal of time at Nazareth Convent, where the Sisters always kept a room for priests who needed quiet and space apart. Sister Berchmans Frison, his friend and compatriot, remembered:

When we now remember the last years of his life, when sickness subdued his ardent spirit and made him long for peace and rest; when he would glide by like a shadow, bent, silent and exhausted...we feel a wave of sadness and compassion steal over our hearts.[2]

    DeRegge was totally devoted to McQuaid, who called him the last of the old guard. DeRegge ordered that, should he die in Europe, his heart be sent to Rochester.

    A young James O'Hare raises a haughty chin away from the camera. Though he lacked the grace, he was no less loyal to McQuaid than Monsignor DeRegge. He never did warm to the Sisters of St. Joseph and treated them with the same sangfroid that was evident in his dismissal of Mother Stanislaus from St. Mary's Asylum. O'Hare was well known in Rochester ecumenical circles; the arrogance he showed toward the Sisters seemed not to have extended to others, who saw him as "gentle, modest and simple."[4] McQuaid thought the world of him, and suggested his name as Bishop for Syracuse. James O'Hare died in 1889, on his fifty-second birthday. Bishop McQuaid wept openly and could barely give the eulogy at the funeral. "I feel like an old man," he said, "who has lost the son who had given promise of being the prop of his father's old age...The loss to me is beyond expression."[5]

    Ann O'Connor Leary, no longer young, leans primly on a brocaded chair: small, a birdlike Irish face, her dress somber black (a reminder of young widowhood), her hands tough and gnarled (a reminder of the years as sole support of six young children), her eyes alert and alive with humor.

    There is a wonderful picture in Concordia of Nellie and Bridget (now with the venerable titles of "Mother Josephine" and "Mother Francis Joseph") with an unidentified priest. The Leary girls, grown generously to middle age, huge in voluminous skirts, round and jolly and lapless; the diminutive priest perched between them, legs crossed, holding a book, as if to distract himself from their mountainous presence.

All had not been jolly for them since they left Rochester with their older sister in 1883. Their stories got lost, overshadowed by hers, but clearly she relied on them more than any others. From the start Mother Stanislaus had given positions of authority to her sisters, to the dismay of Father Dominic, their first mentor and official "spiritual father" in Kansas. He told Bishop Fink that he was "not in favor that sisters of blood have charge of everything" when he heard that Francis Joseph would be left as superior in Newton.[6].

But it was they who Mother Stanislaus sent far and wide to establish the community's presence throughout the west: opening missions in Wisconsin, Nebraska, Texas, and Kansas, Most often they were the superiors of these new missions. Even if the appointments smacked of nepotism, there is no discounting their influence on the spreading reputation of the community and their zeal for quality education in the new West. There must have been restless blood in the Leary line.

They all ended up in LaGrange, in a perfect denouement that could rival any dramatist's design. But the plan, as it played out, was not so perfect. After Mother Stanislaus' death and their refusal to accept Alexine as their superior, they tried to found still another community in Belvidere, Illinois. They evidently lacked their elder sister's talent for founding, because in a few years they were back on Concordia's doorstep, asking to be readmitted. They were accepted and lived to a mellow old age in Kansas.

In the center of the board are the faces of the main players: Father James Early, Bishop Bernard McQuaid and Mother Stanislaus Leary.

Early is older in this picture, his gray hair balding, his bad eyes squinting, lines of pain on his forehead. He hardly looks the jovial young activist who had attracted so many people to himself, or the strong antagonist who had kept McQuaid on edge for fourteen years. It is hard to imagine that this soft, paunchy, baggy-eyed man could be the same "black-horned devil" that Sister Augustine Humphrey had warned the new Bishop about twenty years before. Age is a wonderful leveler.

He and Mother Stanislaus had been friends for so long, had been young together, had joined their zeal in caring for the orphans, had fought McQuaid as a common adversary, though on separate battlefields. She had learned, as friends do, to mirror his strength and wiliness; he had taught her some of the ways of the business world, and encouraged her to trust her own lights.

There are two pictures of Bernard McQuaid One is as he was in his early forties: caught in a noble Napoleonic pose, eyes glancing upwards as though he saw a fine vision. This is the McQuaid that Mother Stanislaus first knew. Strong he looks, and confident. His eyes do not have the tight sternness of later years, though his mouth is already dragged down in a look of permanent disapproval. The second is more typical: full regalia, staff, scowling, looking as though he could never be satisfied.

These pictures reveal nothing of the wit and humanity that often came through in his correspondence, nor of the down-to-earth, avuncular qualities that mark many of his spiritual conferences. As the years went by and time drifted farther and farther from the painful days of the early 1880s, he tightened his grip again on the community and squeezed work and affection from them equally.

In 1903 Abbe Felix Klein, a professor from the Catholic Institute of Paris, visited McQuaid, who took him to "his" Normal School (entirely paid for and supported by the Sisters of St. Joseph, though he would have found that sort of detail trifling). Abbe Klein wrote of that visit:

Nothing I have seen is so thoroughly American as this old man of eighty years, straight, thick-set, vigorous, with a frank and resolute bearing...'I am going to show you my Normal School for Sisters...When I founded this diocese in 1868...there were eight poor Sisters of St. Joseph here. I adopted them as a diocesan congregation. Today there are four hundred. I get whatever service I desire from them without having to apply to distant superiors...You are going to see how they work!'[7]

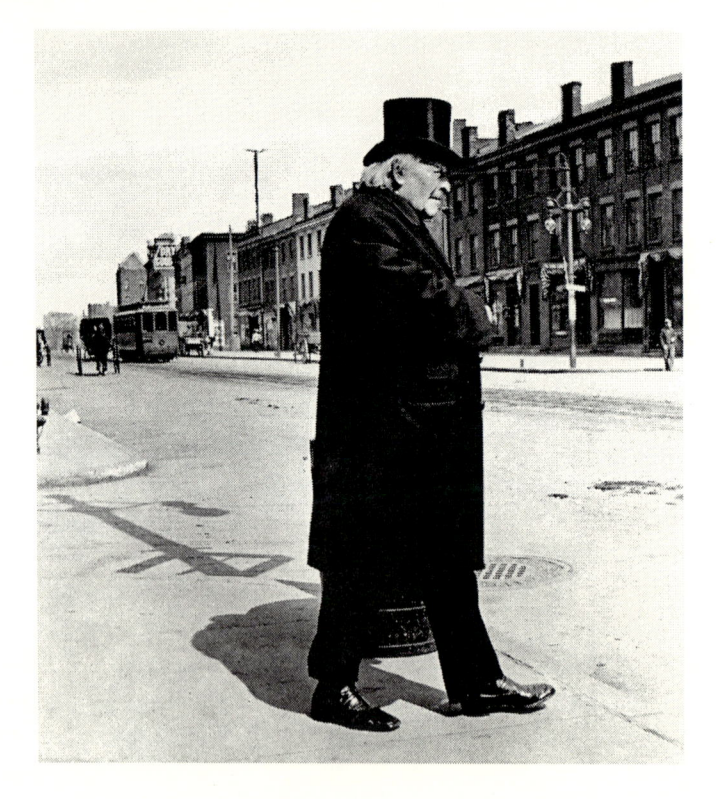

Bishop Bernard McQuaid strolls downtown Rochester

McQuaid took the Abbe on a tour of the Normal School, to show off his nuns. Klein continued:

> In every room that we pass through...the Bishop is welcomed with evident joy. In his own blunt way he scatters jokes, counsel, and when requested, a brief blessing: 'God bless you, God bless you!' One feels that at a sign from him these good Sisters would be ready to fling themselves into the fire and he knows it.[8]

There is no reason to doubt that this was true. Katherine Conway, in her memoir on Bishop McQuaid wrote:

> Sometimes it might have seemed in his dealings with his religious as if he saw chiefly the community and scarcely the individual. But his friends knew better. How he boasted of its membership! The Sisters knew in what esteem he held Mother Agnes: 'She who never put an obstacle in the way of the work, who never told me an untruth, who never brought to me a complaint.'[9]

The implied comparison was transparent. Mother Agnes Hines knew how to handle Bishop McQuaid. He knew he could count on her loyalty, obedience and, eventually, friendship. His letters to her reveal an easy casualness that he never had with Mother Stanislaus.

By the time he died in January 1909, Mother Agnes had established her community as a strong, essential force in the diocese and herself as a capable leader. She had carefully locked the door that led to Kansas; she had succeeded in blocking out the past and in creating a new community. It was as though Mother Stanislaus had never been there. No one talked about those days any more. The "defectors" were long gone; the remaining dissenters, like Sister Adelaide Carberry, were somehow silenced on the subject.

A month after McQuaid died (and nine years after

the death of Mother Stanislaus), Mother Alexine Gosslein wrote to Mother Agnes from LaGrange, asking her to fill in some details about the circumstances surrounding Mother Stanislaus' leaving Rochester, and to provide some information on the early missions Mother Stanislaus had started. The LaGrange community was only nine years old and she wanted to be sure to preserve their history. Though Mother Stanislaus had told her a bit of the real story, she wanted to hear about it from the source.

Mother Agnes had so successfully obliterated the memories of that time that she was able to write back:

February 24, 1909
Dear Mother Alexine,
We send you this condensed extract from our annals of the subsequent life of Mother Stanislaus. You may know more than we do; as also you may have heard accounts of her leaving here, though these events, undoubtedly directed by Providence, have been variously interpreted.

Our annals merely mention the change, without trying to unravel the causes thereof, which very few, if any, seem to have understood rightly. At present very few remember them; but all who have known the kind heart of Mother Stanislaus honor and revere her memory...

Of the schools and convents opened during the administration of Mother Stanislaus, very little now remains as it was in her time; being all diocesan or parish property, with the exception of Nazareth Convent, those places have nearly all been remodeled, enlarged, changed to other sites or demolished. Of the history of those schools very little can be said as they were all in their beginning, struggling to get a start and to overcome the prejudice of the people, the majority of whom were in favor of public schools. Those times have changed.

We have no pictures of any of those schools or convents. Hoping that this writing will be of some use to you,
I remain dear Mother Alexine,
Sincerely yours in C.J.
Mother M. Agnes[10]

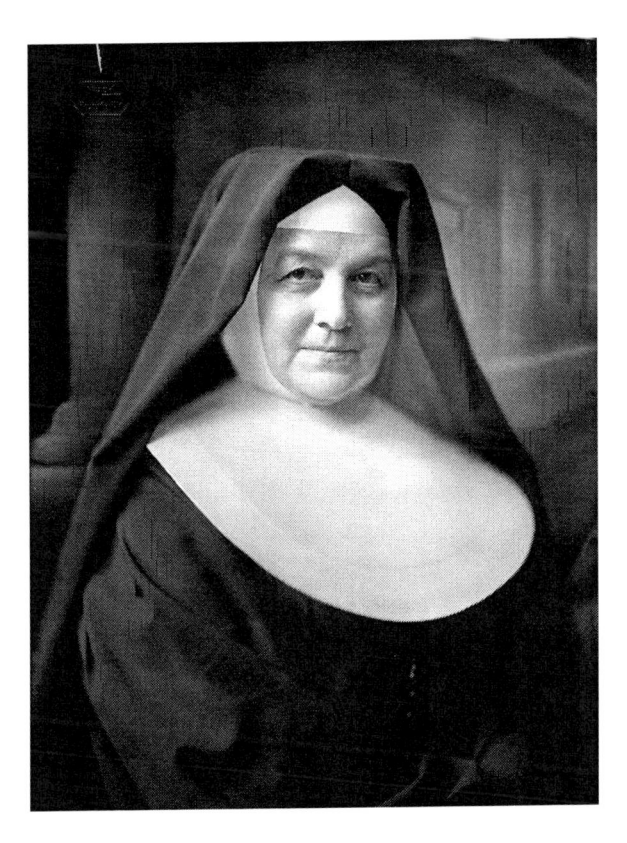

Mother Agnes Hines remained Superior General for thirty-nine years.

    This letter is a study in denial: No one understood, she says, and few remember the circumstances. In fact, no one was in a better position to understand than she; and if she forgot, she had a remarkably selective memory. Some of the Sisters from the eighties lived well into the 1920s. There were many around in 1909: Paul Geary knew; Adelaide knew; Ursula knew; Rose Hendrick knew; Berchmans certainly knew.
    There are no pictures, she says, of the earliest

schools and convents. In fact, pictures of at least nine of the fourteen missions opened by Mother Stanislaus still remain; if anything, there would have been *more* in 1909.

Little is known, she says, of the early history of those missions. In fact, the Annals contain details of each mission as it was established, accounts both factual and anecdotal.

The people resisted the opening of Catholic schools, she says. In fact, the Catholic people welcomed parish schools and had great pride in them. These schools grew very rapidly. McQuaid sometimes had to convince his pastors of their worth, but rarely the parents. It was the good groundwork done during Mother Stanislaus' time that opened the way for the schools that followed.

Was it ignorance or deceit, naiveté or denial, protection of family secrets or selective memory? It is clear that Mother Agnes, for whatever reason, simply did not want to share any of the information with the young LaGrange community. Someone was bound to come out looking bad. Let sleeping dogs lie.

Still, it is a troubling letter. On my board its subject, Mother Stanislaus, eyes slightly averted from the camera, strong, frank, and ordinary. In some ways she is typical of strong women religious of the late 1800s, whose troubles with bishops, problems with finances, and disagreements within their communities forced them to move about, new foundations branching as they passed - women with a simple faith, an uncanny vision, a strong work ethic and sand in their shoes.[11]

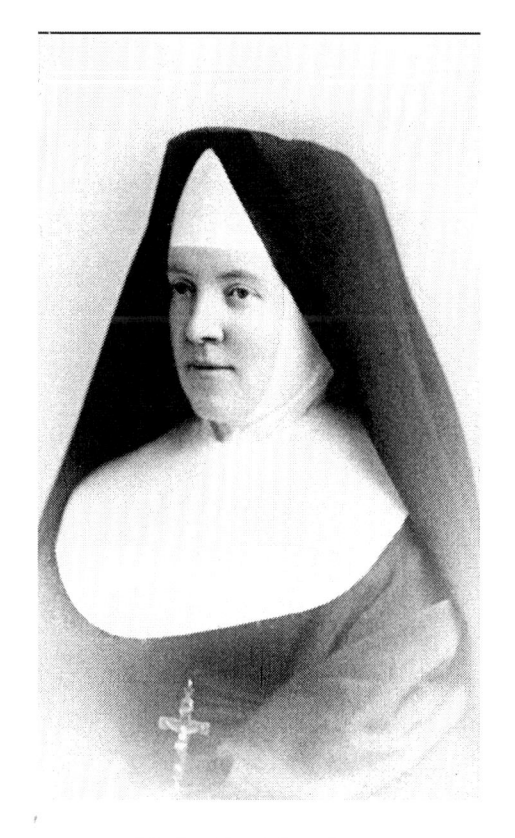

Mother Stanislaus Leary

  She had grown up with the Rochester church and had outgrown it. She had been oblivious of the feminist movement in her midst but had achieved her own liberation. She had gone from softness and subservience to survival and self-reliance. And she had taken so many on her way.
  Eventually another new community of Sisters of St. Joseph spun off from the foundation in LaGrange to Orange, California, making Mother Stanislaus Leary directly or indirectly instrumental in the founding of five independent religious congregations in the United States.

The images flip in rapid succession. Corning, Canandaigua, James Early, her orphans, Seraphine's ravaged face, Baptista, a Hemlock sunset, rows of schoolchildren, ledger books, dying young sisters, Bernard McQuaid, harsh words, flurries of letters, unforgiving hurts, a mystery mansion, the frontier, the betrayal of friends, moving, moving on again, the turning century, the last hours, the release from pain, the footprints left behind.

Whatever the imperfections, pettiness, subterfuge, arrogance, or mistakes that marked the events of those years; however stubborn, authoritarian, secretive and wily she may have become, the power of her sheer goodness, the strength of her simple faith, and the steady vision she was able to maintain gave her an influence that ripples into the twenty-first century.

The heart sees only one continuous movement, one single moment, one enduring grace, one persistent vision.

Key to Abbreviations

ACSJB	Archives Sisters of St. Joseph Brentwood
ACSJC	Archives of St. Joseph Concordia
ACSJL	Archives of St. Joseph LaGrange
ACSJP	Archives of St. Joseph Philadelphia
ACSJW	Archives of St. Joseph Wichita
ASSJB	Archives Sisters of St. Joseph Buffalo
ASSJR	Archives Sisters of St. Joseph Rochester
BDA	Buffalo Diocesan Archives
RDA	Rochester Diocesan Archives
NYAA	New York Archdiocesan Archives

Notes to Chapter 1   Ready for Anything

1. Sister Francis Joseph Ivory, unpublished memoir, copy in ASSJR, p. 10.
2. Bishop John Timon to Mother St. John Fornier, March 29, 1865. Original ACSJP.
3. Bishop John Timon to Mother St. John, June 22, 1856. Original ACSJP.
4. Rev. Edmond O'Connor to Mother St. John, August 4, 1856. Original ACSJP.
5. Bishop John Timon, Letter of Obedience, August 12, 1856. Original ACSJP.

Notes to Chapter 2   A Question of Power

1. There are so many discrepancies in the records and available accounts of Margaret Leary's birth, entrance, reception and profession that it seems best to deal with it at the outset and let it rest. According to books by Sr. Evangeline Thomas and Rev. Robert McNamara as well as records of the Sisters of St. Joseph of LaGrange and Rochester, she was born in 1841. Her own diary contradicts this: "I was born in 1843..." but this could be a lapse of memory on her part. LaGrange records say she died February 14/00, aged 58, so this would make

her birth date to be August 15, 1841. Other dates as they are variously recorded are:

Entrance into the Sisters of St. Joseph:
10/15/57	Rochester
10/15/58	Concordia
1856	Buffalo
10/15/57	LaGrange

Reception of the habit:
2/14/58	Rocheser/ LaGrange
2/14/59	Concordia
2/15/57	Buffalo

Profession of vows:
4/27/60	Rochester
8/15/61	Concordia/ LaGrange
4/27/59	Buffalo

The Buffalo records seem to be the most accurate, since the reception and profession documents are written in her own hand and witnessed.

2. We can only piece together details of the Leary family. It seems there were five girls: Margaret, Nellie and Bridget became Sisters of St. Joseph; Mary Leary married John Donovan and lived in Auburn; Isabelle Leary married a Mr. Matthews and lived in Rochester. Mother Stanislaus mentions a brother in a letter to Bishop McQuaid and notes in her diary that her brother from Montana stopped to visit her in Concordia on his way to Peru in 1889. There is a Dennis Leary who was married at St. Mary's Corning in the 1850s, so this might be he. There are no extant records of Michael Leary's death, but he must have died between August 1848 (when Nellie was conceived) and December 1849 (when the first Corning census was taken).

3. Uri Mulford, *Pioneer Days and Later Times in Corning and Vicinity,* 1789-1920, printed and published by Uri Mulford (Corning, no date), p.202.

4. *Rite of Profession and Reception*, Sisters of St. Joseph. ASSJR.

5. Act of Profession, ASSJB.
6. *Annals* Sisters of St. Joseph of Rochester, Book I, p. 19. ASSJR.
7. St. Mary's Academy was typical of the convent academies of that day: a boarding school for young ladies in which the curriculum was geared toward educating "accomplished" young ladies." Besides the basics of the three R's, they studied the arts and domestic sciences such as embroidering; French was the usual foreign language studied and the girls at St. Mary's were fortunate to have some native French Sisters to teach them.
8. Bishop John Timon to Mother St. John, October 4, 1858. Original in ACSJP.
9. Bishop John Timon to Mother St. John, January 7, 1859. Original in ACSJP.
10. Bishop John Timon, Diary Vol. November 1857-1859. Original in BDA; copy RDA.
11. Bishop John Timon to Mother St. John, June 16, 1859. Original ACSJP.
12. Bishop John Timon to Mother St. John, March 8, 1860. Original ACSJP.
13. Bishop John Timon to Mother St. John, July 18, 1860. Original ACSJP.
14. Bishop John Timon to Mother St. John, June, 1862. Original ACSJP.

Notes to Chapter 3   No Doubt of the Needs

1. cf Ruth Rosenberg-Napersteck, "Life and Death in Nineteenth Century Rochester," *Rochester History,* Vol. XLV, January and April 1983, p. 3.
2. *Ibid*, quoted p. 19.
3. *Ibid*, p. 18.
4. Mary Florence Sullivan, RSM, *Mercy Comes to Rochester,* Sisters of Mercy, Rochester: 1985, p. 46. The controversy over caring for boys was not a new one.

In St. Louis and later in Philadelphia the Sisters of St. Joseph were asked to take charge of boys' asylums when other congregations, whose rules prohibited care of boys, had to abandon them. The rule of the Sisters of St. Joseph had no specific prohibition against caring for boys, though there was never a clear precedent. This left them free to teach both sexes in parochial schools as well, and indeed to take up any work a bishop or pastor might ask of them. This flexibility was a strong factor in the growth of the congregation in the United States. cf. Patricia Byrne CSJ, "Sisters of St. Joseph, the Americanization of a French Tradition," *U.S. Catholic Historian* 5, 1986, p. 110.
5. Sister Augustine Humphrey to Bishop Bernard McQuaid, June 24, 1869. RDA.
6. Teresina Hayes SSJ, *The Sisters of St. Joseph in the Diocese of Rochester*, unpublished ms. p. 58. ASSJR.
7. *Union and Advertiser,* unsigned editorial, Jan. 16, 1865.
8. Rev. Daniel Moore, *Union and Advertiser*, Jan. 26, 1861.
9. Humphrey, op. cit.

Notes to Chapter 4   The Best and Ablest of Friends

1. Sister Mary Agnes Sharkey, *The New Jersey Sisters of Charity*, New York: 1933, I:156.
2. Rev. Daniel Hudson, *Ave Maria*, June 30, 1909; quoted by Katherine Conway, "Memoir of Bishop Bernard McQuaid," unpublished mss, ASSJR, p. 20.
3. Bishop McQuaid to Bishop Corrigan, July 18, 1868; quoted by Frederick Zwierlein, *The Life and Letters of Bishop McQuaid*, Vol II, The Art Print Shop, Rochester: 1926, p. 7.
4. For a full discussion of this, cf Sullivan, *Mercy Comes to Rochester.* op. cit.
5. According to the 1867 *Constitutions:* "The Sisters of the

congregation shall consider the Bishops of the respective dioceses in which they reside as their Superiors: they shall show them profound respect, submission and obedience in all things which they may prescribe, considering them as holding the place of Jesus Christ, and invested with his authority over them. The Bishops can visit the houses of this community established in their respective dioceses and demand an account, both of the temporal and spiritual state of their houses; they can examine, correct, and even punish, according as prudence and charity may suggest to them. They can make regulations for the general good; and for the maintenance and execution of the present Constitutions. They can also, if they deem it useful or necessary, change Superiors and Sisters from one house to another, and even send them to other dioceses, where they are demanded or for other purposes consistent with the object of this community. When any Superiors or Sisters in office desire to renounce their charge, or when it is found necessary to depose them, the Bishop can do so, and name others in their place." *Constitutions of the Congregation of the Sisters of St. Joseph,* McLaughlin Brothers, Philadelphia: 1867, p. 76.

6. These Sisters remained in the Rochester diocese. Dates are entrance dates:

Sister Stanislaus Leary	1856
Augustine Humphrey	1857
Xavier Delahunty	1859
DePazzi Bagley	1862
Ambrose McKeagan	1863
Ignatius Hanlon	1863
Clare O'Shea	1864
Claver Hennessey	1865
Patrick Walsh	unknown
Michael Brown	1865
James O'Connell	1865

      Camillus Payne   1866
      Paul Geary   1866
      Lucy Gorman   1867

7. An old journal in ASSJB (probably written by Mother Mary Ann Burke) recounts this time: "The orphaned condition of the Diocese, the loss of the Sisters to us remaining in Rochester, the mental strain of the new work with new people, the being responsible for so many Sisters and houses all combined to shatter M. Anastasia's constitution, which at best was never robust...After two years of worry and anxiety she was forced to beg of Rt. Rev. Bishop Ryan to accept her resignation, much to the regret of all who knew her sincere, upright, zealous character...She rested then for some months away from all responsibility." p. 84-85.
8. Mother Stanislaus to Bishop McQuaid, April 7, 1870. RDA.
9. *Rochester Daily Advertiser*, October 2, 1848.
10. Mother Stanislaus to Bishop McQuaid, April 7, 1870, op. cit.
11. *Ibid.*
12. Rev. James Early to Bishop McQuaid, May 11, 1870. RDA
13. cf letter of Sister Augustine Humphrey, June 24, 1869. RDA and Rev. James Dougherty, *Diamond Jubilee St. Mary's Church of Canandaigua, New York, 1844-1919*, p. 9. (Financial statements verify the struggle for wages for Sister-teachers.)
14. *Annals*, Vol. I, ASSJR, p. 45.
15. Sister Ignatius Hanlon to Bishop McQuaid, November 4, 1885. RDA.
16. *Ibid.*
17. *Ibid.*
18. *Ibid.*

Notes to Chapter 5   The Old Balancing Act

1. *Rochester and the Post Express: A History of the City of Rochester from Earliest Times*, Post Express Printing Co., undated.
2. *Book of Minutes*, St. Patrick's Asylum, 1870-1882, ASSJR.
3. *West End Journal,* September 1870, p. 1-2. RDA.
4. Minutes, op. cit.
5. *Annals*, Vol. I, p. 47.
6. Teresina Hayes, SSJ, p. 82.
7. *Annals,* Vol. I, p. 47.

Notes to Chapter 6   Ordinary Time

1. These schools were opened during Mother Stanislaus' administration:

Nazareth Academy	1871
Cathedral School	1871
Immaculate Conception	1873
St. Mary, Auburn	1873
St. Rose, Lima	1875
Holy Trinity, Webster	1879
St. Francis de Sales, Geneva	1875
St. Bridget	1875
St. Agnes, Avon	1876
Nativity BVM, Brockport	1876
St. Mary, Dansville	1877
St. Patrick, Seneca Falls	1879

There was also a school attached to each of the orphan asylums.

2. The schools staffed by the Sisters of Mercy during this time were: St. Mary's, where they had been since their arrival in Rochester, Holy Family in Auburn, and Holy

Cross in Rochester, which they took over when the pastor threatened to close the school if the Sisters of Mercy were not hired there.
3. *Jubilee Annals*, p. 87 ASSJR.
4. cf McQuaid, eulogy for Mother Hieronymo and various conferences given to Sisters at Nazareth Convent, collected at ASSJR.
5. During the years 1872-1889, 89 new (or new provinces of) religious congregations were established in the United States. cf Angelyn Dries. "The Americanization of Religious Life," *U.S. Catholic Historian,* Vol. 10, numbers 1 & 2, 1989, p. 22.
6. Jenny Marsh Parker, *Rochester, A Story Historical*, Scrantom and Whitmore, Rochester: *1884, p. 264*-265.
7. Sisters of St. Joseph, *Book of Customs*, handwritten, probably 1864-1899, III: 6, ASSJR.
8. *Ibid,* IV:3.
9. *Jubilee Annals*, p. 96-97.
10. *Annals,* Vol. I, p. 117.
11. The annals and other records give a little information about these early deaths:

Sr. Agatha Kelly, a teacher of the small children at Cathedral School, died of a "sudden and brief but painful illness" in July 1874. She was 20 years old, the first of several novices to make "deathbed professions."

Sr. deSales Corcoran was a Canandaigua girl who taught in the boys' department at Cathedral. She was only sick for two weeks before she died in 1875. She was 23.

Sr. Ignatius Buckley entered the community in January 1875, received the habit in May and died of typhoid pneumonia on September 27.

Sr. Philip Salmon was a lay Sister who worked with the orphan girls at St. Patrick's Asylum. She died in 1876 in the fifth year of her religious life.

Srs. Vincentia Salt and Appolonia Gibbon were both novices. Appolonia was 21, suffering in the final stages of tuberculosis. Mother Stanislaus took Vincentia with her to Canandaigua, so that she could be with Appolonia and be there when she made her vows. Appolonia died three months later, but Vincentia, stricken suddenly, died first.

  Sr. Augustine Burby had become a boarder at Nazareth after her mother died. She entered the community when she was 15, and died five years later. She had been a music teacher, and the *Catholic Times* wrote in her obituary: "The sweet virgin was a music teacher at St. Mary's Auburn, but now we hope she attunes her lyre with the heavenly choirs." *Annals*, p. 113.

  Sr. Petronella Haight entered the community at 17. She taught music for two years before she died.

  Sr. Calasanctius Elmore, a lay Sister who was "a remarkable personal beauty," died in the fourth year of her religious life.

  Sr. Isadore O'Brien died of tuberculosis at age 27. The annalist notes that "she observed the rule" and was a hard worker. "Her little check apron was not laid aside until her habit itself." *Annals*, p. 154.

  Sr. Dominic Hickey, a lay novice, died very suddenly at St. Patrick's Asylum.

  Sr. Michael Brown was the first of the original Rochester group to die. Though she had been a religious for only ten years, she was one of the oldest Sisters in the community at that time. Michael had worked faithfully and hard with the boys at St. Mary's Asylum.

12. *Jubilee Annals*, p. 270 ASSJR.
13. For a complete discussion of this controversy, see Zwierlein, op,cit., Vol. II, Chapter XX.
14. This would be consonant with what we know of Stephen Ryan's personality. He was known for his loyalty to his priests. After his death, the editor of the diocesan paper in Buffalo said of him: "He was cautious yet courageous, gentle but strong, fiery still meek...Irascible by nature, so thoroughly had he conquered himself that he succeeded in acquiring the contrary virtue. He knew how to govern

because he had learned to obey...Above all, Bishop Ryan loved his priests...with all of them he sympathized in their hardships and their trials. And when sometimes more in sorrow than in anger, he found it necessary to be stern in rebuke, mercy stayed the uplifted hand that official duty had raised to strike." Rev. Patrick Cronin, *Catholic Union and Times*, August 27, 1903, p. 1.
15. *Book of Minutes*, St. Patrick's Asylum, ASSJR.

Notes to Chapter 7   Days of Miracles

1. Bishop McQuaid, talk given to Sisters of St. Joseph at Nazareth Convent, August 15, 1871. Quoted in *West End Journal*, September 1871, p. 42.
2. *Annals*, Vol. I p. 77.
3. *Ibid*, p. 98
4. *Ibid,* p. 99.
5. Mary Ann Noah, nee Meeks, was a well-known New York actress in the 1830s and 40s. She was married first to actor Frank McClure who worked with her and Edwin Booth in the celebrated Bowry Theater. After McClure died, she married W.G. Noah, a Buffalo merchant. She is mentioned in T. Allston Brown's *A History of the New York Stage*, Vol. I, Benjamin Bloom Inc., New York: 1903, p. 112 and in Noah Ludlow's *Dramatic Life as I Found It,* Benjamin Bloom, New York: 1880, p. 281 and 397. Mrs. Noah died in Rochester in 1888, aged 80.
6. *Annals,* Vol. 1, p. 68.
7. Obituary clipping, undated, unsigned. ASSJR.
8. Pope Leo XIII had recently been elected. Bishop McQuaid was going to Rome for his first ad limina visit with the new pope. It seemed to be McQuaid's custom to remain a long time in Europe when he made these journeys.
9. *Annals,* Vol. 1, p. 144.

10. *West End Journal*, July 1875.
11. Quoted by Zwierlein, op. cit., Vol. II, p. 182. Original letter February 27, 1879, in NYAA.
12. cf Zwierlein, op. cit., Vol. II, p. 185 and *Rochester Evening Express*, April 27, 1879.
13. *Jubilee Annals*, p. 333-334.
14. Mrs. DeVaney to Mother Stanislaus March 27, 1879. RDA.
15. Quoted in Zwierlein, op. cit., Vol. II, p. 209. For a complete discussion of the Egler case, see Zwierlein, II, Chapter XXII.
16. Exerpts from various letters from Sisters of St. Joseph to Bishop McQuaid. Originals are in RDA, copies in ASSJR.
17. Bishop McQuaid to Mother Stanislaus, letter September 1882. RDA.
18. Bishop McQuaid to Archbp. Corrigan, June 4, 1880. Quoted in Zwierlein, op. cit., Vol. II, p. 194.

Notes to Chapter 8   Wholehearted, Unquerying Children

1. *Jubilee Annals*, p. 369.
2. Quoted in *Annals*, Vol I, p. 156.
3. *Jubilee Annals*, p. 371.
4. *Annals*, Vol I, p. 155.
5. *Annals*, Vol. I, p. 159.
6. Mother Stanislaus to Bishop McQuaid, letter January 17, 1881. RDA.
7. According to St. Mary's Asylum records, Nazareth Convent borrowed $2082.08 in 1879; this indebtedness was reduced to $1700 by January 1880. Community records show a loan of $10,843 for mortgage and interest payments in 1879. cf St. Mary's Asylum Minutes, Nazareth Convent Account Book, 1879-87, ASSJR.
8. Mother Stanislaus to Bishop McQuaid, January 20, 1881. RDA.
9. *Annals* I, p. 166

10. In 1884 Katherine Conway joined the staff of the Boston *Pilot* and eventually became its editor.
11. Katherine Conway, "Memoir of Bishop Bernard McQuaid," op. cit., p. 16.
12. Ibid, p. 17.
13. Alice Seymour to Bishop McQuaid, July 18, 1881. RDA.
14. *Ibid.*
15. *Annals,* Vol I, p. 170.
16. *Ibid,* p. 172.
17. *Jubilee Annals*, p. 419.
18. Alice Seymour to Bishop McQuaid, op. cit.
19. *Jubilee Annals*, p. 420.
20. Bishop McQuaid to Mother Stanislaus, December 17, 1881. RDA. According to the 1867 Constitution, "The monitor is appointed to admonish the Superior of her faults and to receive such complaints as may be made against her...When an inferior makes a complaint against the Superior, she shall mildly listen to what is said without, at the same time, giving entire credit to it; and she shall deliberately inquire about the matter with great prudence before she admonishes the Superior...In case of her failure to remedy the matter she shall inform the Spiritual Father of it." *Constitutions of the Sisters of St Joseph*, Philadelphia 1867.

Notes to Chapter 9   For Reasons Best Known to Himself

1. *Annals,* Vol. I, p. 185.
2. According to the 1867 *Constitutions*, the process for admitting candidates to vows was: one month before the profession, the Superior General calls together her council, the Mistress of Novices and any professed Sisters who know the novices and asks them one by one about the novices' fitness for religious life. Then she calls the novices themselves in and questions them. The

novices leave and the Sisters vote. Majority rules. The superior gives the names of those they accepted to the bishop and he in turn interviews them. If he approves, they are admitted to profession.

3. *Annals* I, p. 186.
4. Nazareth Convent ledger records the following traveling expenses: 1/14/82 to New York City and 1/21/82 to Erie.
5. *Ontario Messenger*, undated clipping in ASSJR.
6. *Ibid.*
7. Mother Stanislaus to Bishop McQuaid, April 22, 1882. RDA.
8. cf Council Minutes, June 7, 1882. Sisters of St. Joseph of Rochester.
9. cf Council Minutes, June 5, 1882.
10. cf Sr. Imelda Kryger CSJ LaGrange. Unpublished MSS in ACSJL. Chapter 14.
11. *Annals I*, p. 194-196.
12. Sister Berchmans Frison to Bishop McQuaid, May 17, 1882. RDA.
13. Bishop McQuaid to Mother Stanislaus, May 18, 1882. RDA.
14. *Annals I*, p. 197-198.
15. Bishop McQuaid, sermon 12/29/84. Quoted in *Union Advertiser*, 12/31/84.
16. Conference at Nazareth Convent, August 26, 1899. ASSJR.
17. Conference at Nazareth Convent, August 20, 1889. ASSJR.
18. Katherine Conway, "Memoir of Bp. McQuaid," op. cit.
19. *Ibid.*
20. *Annals* I, p. 194, 199.

Notes to Chapter 10   If You Will Just Leave Me Alone

1. Council Minutes, June 2, 1882. Sisters of St. Joseph of Rochester.
2. Rev. Michael O'Brien to Bishop McQuaid, November

20, 1875. RDA.
3. Council Minutes, June 5, 1882. Sisters of St. Joseph of Rochester.
4. *Ibid.*
5. William F. Gelston to Bishop McQuaid, April 3, 8, 22; June 6; July 18, 1882. RDA.
6. Council Minutes, op. cit.
7. Council Minutes, June 7, 1882. Sisters of St. Joseph of Rochester
8. *Ibid.*
9. Sister Adelaide Carberry to Bishop McQuaid, June 19, 1882. RDA.
10. *The Catholic Union and Times*, June 8, 1882, p. 5. BDA.
11. Sister Delphine CSJ to Bishop McQuaid, June 12, 1882. RDA.
12 Bishop McQuaid to Bishop Ryan, June 15, 1882. RDA.
13. Katherine E. Conway to Bishop McQuaid, August 6, 1886. RDA.
14. Mother Agnes Hines to Bishop McQuaid, June 14, 1882. RDA.
15. Mrs. Matthews was Mother Stanislaus' sister, Isabelle.
16. Rev. James Early to Mother Stanislaus, July 5, 1882. RDA.
17. Mother Stanislaus to Bishop McQuaid, September 6, 1882. RDA.
18. Council Minutes, September 7, 1882. SSJR.
19. *Ibid.*
20. Mother Stanislaus to Bishop McQuaid, September 12, 1882. RDA.
21. Bishop McQuaid to Mother Stanislaus, date illegible, but probably September, 1882. RDA.
22. Council Minutes, October 13, 1882. Sisters of St. Joseph of Rochester
23. Council Minutes, October 13 and 28, 1882. Sisters of St. Joseph of Rochester
24. Sr. Julia Clinton.
25. Council Minutes, December 31, 1882. Sisters of St.

26. Bishop McQuaid to Mother Stanislaus, February 23. 1883. RDA.
27. It is curious to note that, though the letter to Bishop Fink is signed "Sr. Ursula," it is definitely written in Mother Stanislaus' handwriting! For some reason she felt she could or should not be the direct correspondent.

Notes to Chapter 11   They Are Not Here

1. Council Minutes, December 1, 1882. Sisters of St. Joseph of Rochester
2. Council Minutes, November 18, 1882. Sisters of St. Joseph of Rochester
3. Council Minutes, April 19, 1882. Sisters of St. Joseph of Rochester
4. Mother Stanislaus Leary, Diary and Book of Records, handwritten. ACSJC.
5. Council Minutes, July 31, 1883, September 22, 1883. Sisters of St. Joseph of Rochester
6. "S.M.B.," handwritten notes for annals, September 4, 1884, Vol. 1B (1864-1894) author unnamed. ASSJR.
7. *Annals*, Vol. II, p. 12-13. ASSJR.
8. Felix Swemberg had acted for many years as a colonization agent for the Santa Fe railroad. He started St. Mary's Church in Newton in 1871, with four families, holding services in a tent, in a Santa Fe bunk car, in family homes. By the time the Sisters arrived, he was well established and set in his ways. cf. William Moran, *The Santa Fe and the Chisolm Trail at Newton, Kansas: Centennial Booklet*, 1971, p. 85-86.
9. *Ibid*, p. 79.
10. Richard White, *It's Your Misfortune and None of My Own. A New History of the American West*, University of Oklahoma Press Norman: 1991, p. 309.
11. *Diary*, op. cit. As it turned out, Mother Stanislaus was a

good judge of character and wise to have been leery of Father Swemberg. In 1886 Bishop Fink wrote to Bishop McQuaid, warning him of Swemberg's suspension "for crimes that have come to light of late" and the possibility that Swemberg might apply to Rochester with forged credentials. cf Letter from Bp. Fink to McQuaid, June 1, 1886. RDA.
12. *Ibid.*
13. *Ibid.*
14. Rev. Dominic Meier to Bishop McQuaid, April 26, 1884. RDA.
15. Mother Stanislaus to Bishop McQuaid, May 25, 1884. RDA.
16. Council Minutes, August 2, 1884. Sisters of St. Joseph of Rochester.

Notes to Chapter 12   What the Past Has Made Us

1. C. Robert Haywood, *Victorian West: Class and Culture in Kansas Cattle Towns*, University of Kansas Press, Lawrence: 1991, p. 61.
2. Mary deZeng to Mother Stanislaus, April 23 (year unknown, but probably 1883), orig. ACSJC.
3. *Ibid.*
4. Mother Stanislaus to Bishop Louis Fink, February 7, 1884. ACSJC.
5. Mother Stanislaus Leary, Diary, 1889. ACSJC.
6. *The City of the Plains: Abilene*, Burdett Co., Burlington, IA: 1887, reprinted by Dickinson County Historical Society, 1976. pp. 23, 61, 51.
7. *Ibid*, p. 50.
8. Sr. Madeline Perry CSJ (Concordia), interview October 12, 1938. ACSJC.
10. cf interview Sr. Victoria Lake CSJWA, no date. Files of Sister Eileen Quinlan CSJ (Wichita). According to Sister Eileen "As the years passed, the two communities have accepted their early history and today they work together to carry out their common mission."

11. Mother Stanislaus Leary, <u>Diary</u>, 1889. ACSJC.
12. *Ibid.*
13. Rev. Peter Colgan to Bishop McQuaid, February 18, 1890. RDA.
14. Sister Mary Catherine Monaghan, RSM.
15. Rev. Peter Colgan to Bishop McQuaid, March 5, 1890. RDA.
16. Original telegram ACSJC.
17. Mother Antoinette Cuff, "Recollections of Mother Antoinette Cuff of her Life in the Community," unpublished interview, circa 1925. ACSJC.

Notes to Chapter 13   The Dust From My Feet

1. Mother Stanislaus to Mother Clement, March 15 and April 2, 1897. ACSJC.
2. cf. exchange of letters between Mother Clement and Mother Stanislaus; Mother Clement and Fr. Sabetti, February-March 1898, ACSJC.
3. Sister Isabelle Poisson CSJ (Concordia), interviewed by Sister Emmanuela O'Malley, June 1975. ACSJC.
4. *Ibid.*
5. cf. St. Mary's Asylum Minutes, Nazareth Convent Account Book, 1879-1887, ASSJR.
6. Poisson, op. cit.
7. *Ibid.*
8. *Ibid.*
9. Sister Evelyn Fraser CSJ (Concordia). Interviewed by Sr. Emmanuela O'Malley 4/30/82. ACSJC.
10. Kryger, op. cit., p. 114.
11. *Annals,* Sisters of St. Joseph of LaGrange, not paginated.
12. Frasier, op. cit.

Notes to Chapter 14   In A Borrowed Grave

1. Kryger, Chapter 23
2. Clipping in ASSJR; undated obituary, no author.
3. Teresina Hayes, SSJ, op. cit. p. 271.

4. In 1914, Mother Stanislaus' remains were transferred to Mt. Carmel Cemetery. Mother Alexine Gosslein directed that her headstone read: "Mother Mary Stanislaus Leary, Foundress."
5. Jane Ellen Egan to Mother Alexine Gosslein, February 10, 1901, ACSJL.
6. Monsignor J.E. Leberge to Mother Alexine Gosslein, December 3, 1900, ACSJL.
7. Kryger, Chapter 21.

Notes to Collage: The Rest of the Picture

1. Original picture ACSJL.
2. *Annals* III, p. 23. ASSJR.
3. Rev. James O'Hare to Bishop McQuaid, 1889 (no month noted). RDA.
4. Newspaper clipping, undated, unsigned. ASSJR.
5. *Ibid.*
6. Rev. Dominic Meier to Bishop Fink, August 12, 1884. Kansas Catholic Historical Society. Quoted in Thomas, p. 144.
7. Felix Klein, *In the Land of the Strenuous Life*, A.C. McClurg and Co., Chicago: 1905, pp. 96-104; 112-113; quoted in *Documents of American Catholic History,* ed. John Tracy Ellis, Bruce, Milwaukee: 1962, p. 547.
8. *Ibid.*
9. Conway, "Memoir of Bishop McQuaid" op. cit. p. 47.
10. Mother Agnes Hines SSJ to Mother Alexine Gosslein CSJ, February 24, 1909. ACSJL. Though it is signed by Mother Agnes, this letter is written in the hand of Sister Berchmans Frison, the writer of the *Annals.*
11. I owe this term to Sister Margaret Quinn, Archivist for CSJ Brentwood, who told me that often those Sisters "with sand in their shoes" would come to St. John's Home in Brooklyn (where Sr. Baptista Hanson was long the superior) before going on to found new places.

Works Consulted

Primary Sources:

Letters from Rochester Diocesan Archives, Archives of Sisters of St. Joseph of: Rochester, Philadelphia, Brentwood, Concordia, Wichita, LaGrange

Financial records, receipts, deeds: Rochester Diocesan Archives and Sisters of St. Joseph of Rochester

Community records of Sisters of St. Joseph of Rochester, Buffalo, Concordia

Council Minutes of Sisters of St. Joseph of Rochester

Book of Minutes, St. Mary's Boys' Orphan Asylum, 1865-1890, SSJRA

St. Mary's Asylum Minutes, 1879-1887 ASSJR

Nazareth Convent Account Book, 1879-1887 ASSJR

Book of Customs, Sisters of St. Joseph of Rochester, handwritten, probably 1864-1899, ASSJR

Formulary of Prayers for the Use of the Sisters of St. Joseph, P. O'Shea, New York: 1882

. *Constitution of the Sisters of St. Joseph*, McLaughlin, Philadelphia: 1867, 189 pp. ASSJR

Annals of the Sisters of St. Joseph of Rochester, ASSJR

Jubilee Annals of the Sisters of St. Joseph, 1894, ASSJR

Diary and *Book of Records,* Mother Stanislaus Leary, handwritten ACSJC

Diary, Bishop John Timon,, transcribed by Leonard Reforgiato. Original in BDA, copy in RDA

Historical notes, from 1854-1913, probably by Mother Mary Ann Burke, handwritten, ASSJB

Census records: Geneva Historical Society, Rundell Memorial Library, Rochester, National Archives

Newspapers:

Rochester *Post-Express, West End Journal, Evening Express, Union and Advertiser*

Buffalo *Catholic Union and Times*

Canandaigua *Ontario Messenger*

Unpublished manuscripts and memoirs:

Connaughton, Maureen, *Journeys Begun: The History of the Sisters of St. Joseph LaGrange, Illinois 1830-1930,* unpublished manuscript in ACSJL

Cuff, Mother Antoinette, "Historical Reminiscences of the Sisters of St. Joseph and their Early History in Kansas" ACSJC

Conway, Katherine, "Memoir of Bishop Bernard McQuaid," unpublished manuscript, undated ASSJR

Hayes, Sr. Teresina, SSJ, *The Sisters of St. Joseph in the Diocese of Rochester*, 2 volumes, ASSJR

U.S. Federation of the Sisters of St. Joseph Research Project, oral history transcripts, ACSJC

Books:

Beales, Irene. *Genesee Valley Women 1743-1985,* Chestnut Hill Press, Geneseo: 1985, 223 pp.

Deuther, Charles G. *The Life and Times of the Rt. Rev. John Timon,* published by the author, Buffalo: 1870.

Dolan, Jay P. *The American Catholic Experience,* University of Notre Dame Press, Notre Dame: 1992, 504 pp.

Dunne, Sr. M. of the Sacred Heart. *The Congregation of St. Joseph of the Diocese of Buffalo 1854-1933,* The Holling Press, Buffalo: 1934, 169 pp.

Haywood, C. Robert. *Victorian West: Class and Culture in Kansas Cattle Towns,* University of Kansas Press, Lawrence: 1991, 325 pp.

Hurley, L.M. *Newton, Kansas, a Railway Town 1871-1971,* Mennonite Press, Inc., North Newton: 1985, 184 pp.

Long, R.M. *Wichita Century,* The Wichita Museum Association, Wichita: 1969, 272 pp.

McNamara Robert F. *A Century of Grace: The History of St. Mary's Roman Catholic Parish, Corning, New York,* Christopher Press, Rochester: 1948, 282 pp.

_____. *The Diocese of Rochester 1868-1968,* The Christopher Press, Rochester: 1968, 618 pp.

Meany, Sr. Mary Ignatius. *By Railway or Rainbow, A History of the Sisters of St. Joseph of Brentwood,* Pine Press, Brentwood: 1964, 336pp.

McKelvey, Blake. *Rochester on the Genesee,* Syracuse University Press, Syracuse: 1973, 292 pp.

_____. *Rochester the Water Power City 1812-1854,* Harvard University Press, Cambridge: 1945, 383 pp.

Mulford, Uri. *Pioneer Days and Later Times in Corning and Vicinity 1789-1920,* published by author, Corning, no date but probably 1920.

Parker, Jenny Marsh. *Rochester, A Story Historical,* Scrantom and Witmore, Rochester: 1884, 411pp.

Peck, William F. *History of Rochester and Monroe County, Volume 1,* The Pioneer Publishing Company, New York: 1908, 706 pp.

Phillips, David, ed. *The Taming of the West,* Henry Regenery Co., Chicago: 1974, 233 pp.

Quinlan, Sr. Eileen. *Planted on the Plains: A History of the Sisters of St. Joseph of Wichita, Kansas,* published through Greg D. Jones and Associates, Wichita: 1984, 394 pp.

Smith, Sebastian. *Notes on the Second Plenary Council of Baltimore,* New York: 1874.

Stratton, Joanna L. *Pioneer Women: Voices from the Kansas Frontier,* Simon and Shuster, New York: 1981, 319 pp.

Sullivan, Sr. Mary Florence. *Mercy Comes to Rochester,* Sisters of Mercy, Rochester: 1985, 141 pp.

Thomas, Sr. M. Evangeline. *Footprints on the Frontier: A History of the Sisters of St. Joseph Concordia, Kansas,* The Newman Press, Westminster, MD: 1948, 400 pp.

White, Richard. *It's Your Misfortune and None of My Own: A New History of the American West,* University of Oklahoma Press, Norman: 1991, 645 pp.

Zwierlein, Frederick J. *The Life and Letters of Bishop McQuaid,* The Art Print Shop, Rochester: 1926, 3 volumes.

Booklets:

"Centennial Souvenir and Chronological History of Rochester," Post Express Printing Co., Rochester: 1884.

Brennan, Gerald T. "One Hundred Years of Grace: St. Bridget's Church", Christopher Press, Rochester: 1954, 54 pp.

"The City of the Plains: Abilene", Burdett Company, Burkington, IA: 1887, reprinted by Dickinson County Historical Society, 1976.

"Crowning a Century of Progress: Nativity of the Blessed Virgin Mary Parish", Christopher Press, Brockport, NY: 1955.

Dimitroff, Thomas P. and Janes, Lois S. " History of the Corning Painted Post Area: 200 Years in Painted Post Country," Corning Area Bicentennial

Committee, Corning: 1977, 384 pp.

Dougherty, James T. "Diamond Jubilee St. Mary's Church of Canandaigua", New York 1844-1919, 36 pp.

Gleichauf, Pat and Kingston, Maureen. "The History of St. Agnes Church: 120th Anniversary Celebration 1869-1989", Avon, NY: 1989, 23 pp.

"Golden Jubilee Souvenir of the Immaculate Conception Church", The John Smith Printing House, Rochester: 1899, 131 pp.

Hasmer, Howard, "Monroe County 1821-1971, the Sesquicentennial Account of the History of Monroe County, New York", Flower City Printing, Inc.. Rochester: 1971, 327 pp.

"Holy Trinity Centennial Celebration," 1861-1961, Penny Saver Press, Webster, NY: 1961.

Leonard, Margaret Haley. "History of St. Patrick's Parish, Seneca Falls, NY 1831-1979", no publisher, 1979, 127 pp.

Letchworth, William. " Homes of Homeless Children: A Report on Orphan Asylums and Other Institutions for the Care of Children", New York: 1876.

Moran, William T. " Sante Fe and the Chisolm Trail at Newton, Kansas: Centennial Booklet", 1971.

"One Hundred Years 1849-1949: The History of Immaculate Conception Church", Christopher Press, Rochester: 1949, 64 pp.

Rauber, William J. "Parish Pathways 1845-1945", Genesee County Express, Dansville, NY: 1945, 88 pp.

"The Semi-Centennial Souvenir and Chronological History of Rochester", Post Express Printing Co., Rochester: 1884.

Articles:

Dries, Angelyn OSF. "The Americanization of Religious Life 1872-1922," *U.S. Catholic Historian,* Volume 10, Numbers 1 & 2, 1989, p. 13-24.

Byrne, Patricia SSJ. "Sisters of St. Joseph: The Americanization of a French Tradition," *U.S. Catholic Historian* 5, 1986, pp. 241-272.

Ewens, Mary OP. "The Leadership of Nuns in Immigrant Catholicism," *Women and Religion in America, Vol. 1: The Nineteenth Century,* Rosemary Reuther and Rosemary S. Keller, eds., Harper and Row, San Francisco: 1981, pp. 101-149.

Fisher, Donald M. "The Civil War Draft in Rochester, Part II," *Rochester History,* Spring 1991,No.2.

Jarrell, Lynn, O.S.A., J.C.D. "The Development of Legal Structures for Women Religious Between 1500 and 1900: A Study of Selected Institutes of Religious Life for Women," *U.S. Catholic Historian,* Volume 10, Nos. 1 and 2, 1989, p. 25-35.

Kantowicz, Edward, "Schools and Sisters," *Corporation*

Sole, Notre Dame Press, 1983, p. 260-263. In *American Catholic Religious Life,* from *The Heritage of American Catholicism* series, ed. Timothy Garland.

Kolmer, Elizabeth. "Catholic Women Religious and Women's History: A Survey of the Literature," *Women in American Religion,* Janet James, ed., Philadelphia: 1980, 127-139.

Mannard, Joseph. "Maternity...of the Spirit: Nuns and Domesticity in Antebellum America, "*U.S. Catholic Historian* 5, 1986, p. 305-324.

McKelvey, Blake. "Historic Origins of Rochester's Social Welfare Agencies, "*Rochester History,* April 1947, nos. 2 and 3.

_____. "The Irish in Rochester, an Historical Retrospect," *Rochester History,* October 1957, No. 4.

_____. "Rochester's Ethnic Transformation," *Rochester History,* July 1963, No. 3.

Rosenberg-Napersteck, Ruth. "Life and Death in Nineteenth Century Rochester," *Rochester History,* Vol. XLV, January and April, 1983.